SKIN
HEALING
EXPERT

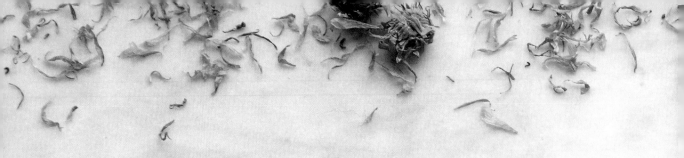

To you, beautiful warrior. Let the journey begin.

An Hachette UK Company
www.hachette.co.uk

First published in Great Britain in 2020 by
Kyle Books, an imprint of Kyle Cathie Ltd
Carmelite House
50 Victoria Embankment
London EC4Y 0DZ
www.kylebooks.co.uk

ISBN: 978 0 85783 8438

Distributed in the US by Hachette Book Group, 1290
Avenue of the Americas, 4th and 5th Floors, New York,
NY 10104

Distributed in Canada by Canadian Manda Group, 664
Annette St., Toronto, Ontario, Canada M6S 2C8

Publisher: Joanna Copestick
Editorial Director: Judith Hannam
Editor: Tara O'Sullivan
Editorial Assistant: Sarah Kyle
Design: Tania Gomes
Photography: Clare Winfield
Food styling: Megan Davies
Props styling: Hannah Wilkinson
Illustrations: Grace Law
Production: Caroline Alberti

A Cataloguing in Publication record for this title is
available from the British Library

Printed and bound in China

10 9 8 7 6 5 4 3 2 1

HC

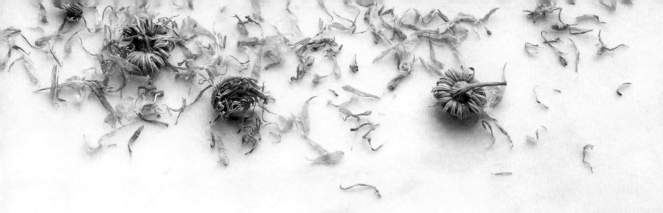

SKIN HEALING EXPERT

Your 5 pillar
plan for calm,
clear skin

HANNA SILLITOE

Photography by Clare Winfield

KYLE BOOKS

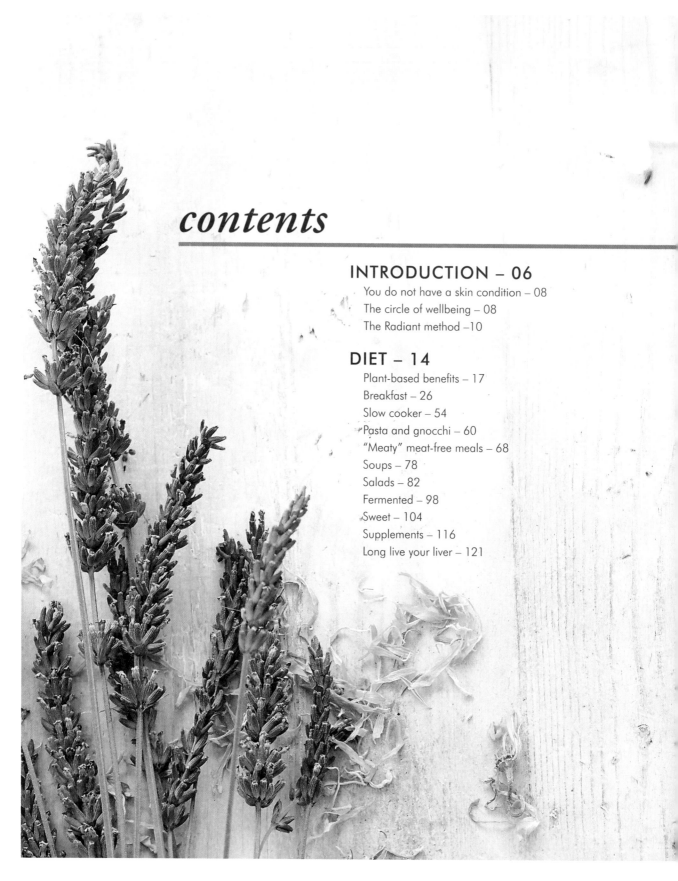

contents

INTRODUCTION – 06

DIET – 14

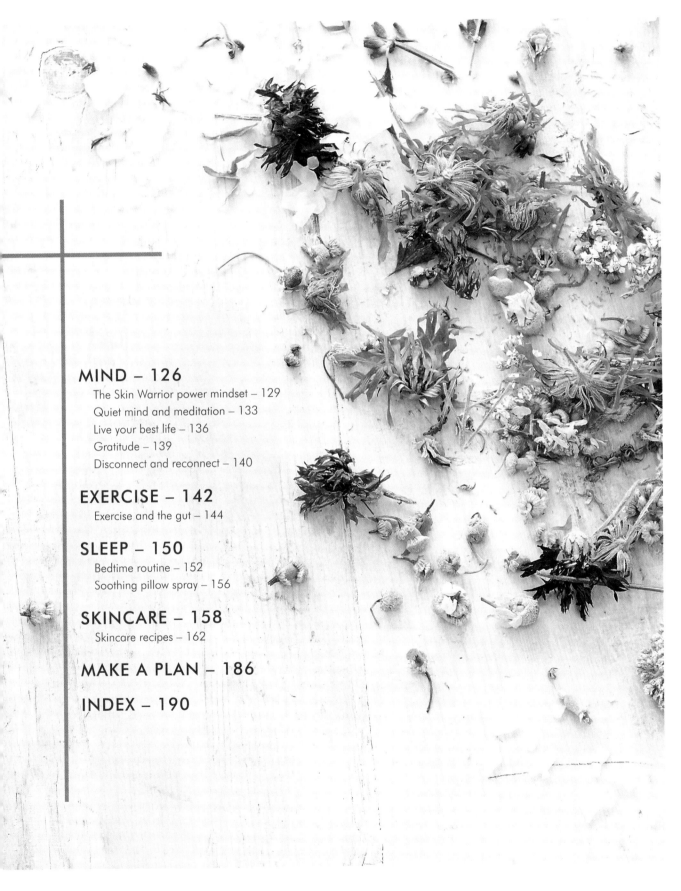

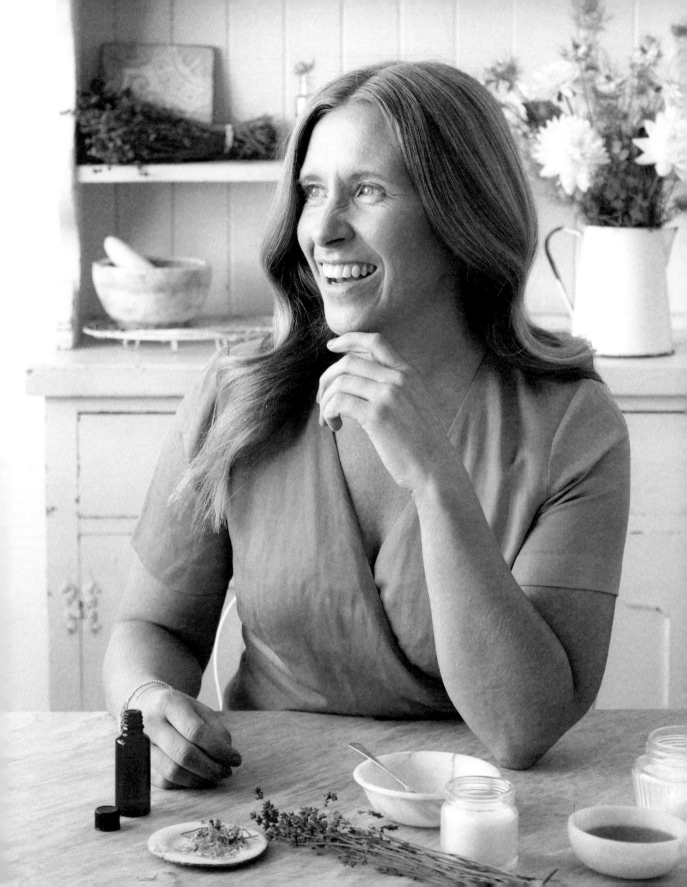

ALL OR *something*

It's been six years since I first began my journey to clear skin. During that time, I've learned a lot about myself, but more importantly, I've learned a great deal from the natural skin-healing community of which I am so proud to be a part.

My skin ruled my life from my teenage years onwards. Acne aged fifteen, my first psoriasis flare right before my high school exams, dry patches of eczema on my face … More than just irritating my skin, these conditions dictated so many aspects of my life. Chronic skin disease is all consuming and exhausting. The joyful things most people take for granted – such as an invitation to a summer party – can fill you with dread, wondering if you can find a summery outfit that will still cover your arms and legs.

I am most definitely an all-or-nothing kind of person. That goes for the bad as well as the good. I remember once hosting a barbecue with my boyfriend. We'd completely run out of alcohol and it was going home time, but I found a half-full bottle of Pimms at the back of the cupboard and insisted on pouring everyone shots at 3am. I didn't want to stop: the party didn't need to end, there always had to be something more.

On the plus side, if I conjure up something positive in my head, I always successfully achieve it, and my dreams can be pretty epic. Not content with participating in my local 5km charity run, I am currently training with an aim to completing an Ironman. This insanely gruelling event incorporates a 2.4-mile swim, a 112-mile bike ride and a marathon. When the thought entered my mind, I hadn't even attempted a short distance triathlon. A year on, I've just successfully completed my first half-Ironman. The full Ironman dream is still very much alive, and I won't stop until I've done it.

When my doctor told me that the next option for trying to treat my skin conditions was a chemotherapy drug, I turned this determination to a complete overhaul of my diet and lifestyle. I quit drinking, smoking and caffeine, and completely changed the way that I ate. This, in turn, healed my skin, and I've been free of psoriasis, acne and eczema ever since.

When it comes to making dietary changes to heal the skin, I realize this all-or-nothing approach can feel a bit too intense for some. My first book, *Radiant*, features a stringent 28-day programme. Embarking on something so strict can be tough and the last thing I want you to feel, simply because my dive-in-feet-first approach doesn't work for you, is failure. There is no such thing as failing when making a tremendous life change. This book is designed to help you build your own step-by-step programme, tailored to best suit you.

We all tread such different paths to reach our final goal. Your route might be slower, but the end result will be the same. Be patient and kind to yourself. This is your journey. Enjoy it, because as daunting as it might feel right now, this really is the start of a brand new, vibrant adventure towards the best health of your life!

YOU DO NOT HAVE A SKIN CONDITION

This might sound like a ridiculous statement. It's certainly something your doctor or dermatologist probably hasn't said. I can sense you're reading this now and screaming, "Of course I've got a skin condition! It's there, it's visible and it's affecting so many different aspects of my life."

To begin treating skin disease differently, we have to begin thinking differently about the underlying triggers. I believe that what you have is a *gut* condition, the symptoms of which are manifesting on the surface of your skin.

If you've seen a doctor or dermatologist about your skin problems, the chances are that you've been prescribed coal tar ointments, acne lotions, or steroid creams at some stage. You'll know that these topical corticoids only ever treat the symptoms. Sometimes you'll apply them and they seem to work like magic; the skin begins to get better, redness fades, pimples disappear, but you stop using them and BOOM, the skin flares up again, sometimes even worse than the first time around. Why? Because you did not resolve the underlying problem – the gut. The gut is a complex little beast. So many factors come into play when considering the happiness of our gut, and this is about so much more than simply eating the right things.

Modern medicine has offered us very targeted relief. We pinpoint where the problem lies and a pill miraculously takes the ailment away. We view ourselves boxed off into all these different little segmented parts, forgetting that all our organs, brain matter, nerve endings, immune system, and skin cells are intrinsically connected. For example, we know that stress isn't good for our health, but we fail to notice the very direct correlation between our mind and our gut. You know that sick feeling in the pit of your stomach when you feel particularly fearful or anxious? Almost as if your stomach is tied in knots – sometimes to the point of not wanting to eat? That's the gut being impacted by the mind.

Seventy per cent of our immune system is housed in our gut and the brain–gut axis is real. When you're stressed, the diversity of microorganisms in your gut is affected. The higher our levels of stress, the more we see our levels of bad bacteria increase and good bacteria decrease, which directly impacts our immune system and, in turn, our skin.

THE CIRCLE OF WELLBEING

Because my brain is so used to being given a set of rules, and rigidly, unwaveringly following them until I've achieved the desired outcome, learning to work with clients who struggle with such a head-strong approach has been a fantastic life lesson. I am often asked if it's possible to heal without following a super-strict detox. Of course. Will it take longer? Possibly, but that's okay, too. On the plus side, this approach can feel much more manageable and practical, which in turn can be key to staying on track.

If something feels incredibly difficult, the temptation to throw in the towel and quit early on is very much there. Through gradually implementing change, there really are no excuses, only foundations that you can continue to build on as you go.

Ill health generally doesn't happen overnight. In the case of your skin flaring up, it might sometimes seem as though it does, but the chances are that for a long time there's been a slow process happening behind the scenes to get you to the point you're at today. Sure, we can talk about the role of genetics but it is usually an accumulation of poor diet and lifestyle, stress and emotional factors that create a full-blown flare.

SWITCH TO A CIRCLE OF WELLBEING

My mission is to make changes from the circle of poor health to strengthen the circle of wellbeing. This doesn't need to be done all at once. You'll notice that as you begin focusing on improving just some of these elements, they, in turn, strengthen others.

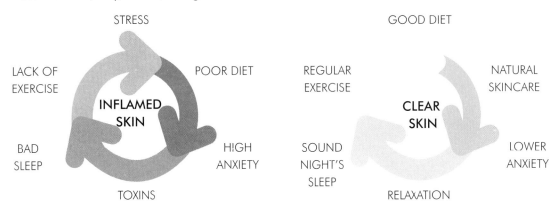

Think of skin disease as a vicious circle – one we're trying to break. Once you start adopting some of the good habits from the circle of wellbeing, you will find those healthy choices begin to build and become second nature. Gradually life will start looking more like the circle of wellbeing.

You'll also find that taking small steps and concentrating on changing just one part of the circle has a positive impact on everything else around it. For example, if you make it your mission in week one to begin exercising each day, you might find you sleep better at night, which in turn helps reduce stress and calm your mind. By beginning with just one change, others soon follow in a snowball effect.

Here are some examples of step-by-step changes you can begin making right away. Choose three to start with one week, then add another three the next week, three the week after, and three the week after that. The changes don't have to be the ones listed. You might want to add your own ideas to the list. Write them down in your journal or scribble them on sticky notes somewhere prominent, and make a commitment to add three new ones each week over the next month to build that circle of wellbeing.

Practise 2-minute daily meditation
Drink 2 litres (3½ pints) of still, fresh water daily
Drink green juice daily
Exercise 15 minutes a day every day
Commit to a regular bedtime routine daily
Switch to natural skincare products

Try a new exercise
Choose a day to focus on meal prep for the week
Drink your herbal tea and take vitamins daily
Set your intentions
Practise gratitude
Commit to three meat-free days this week

THE RADIANT METHOD

If you've read my first book, *Radiant*, you'll know that it features a pretty strict 28-day plan, excluding lots of food groups. I don't want to overwhelm you by giving you a long list of foods to avoid. I'd prefer us to begin by concentrating on all the exciting new juices, recipes and skincare we're going to introduce. That said, there's no getting away from it, there are certain foods that can exacerbate skin problems, so these are ones we'll look to reduce over the coming weeks and months.

Some of these foods are pretty obvious and perhaps ones you've already looked to cut down on or eliminate from your diet. Others, such as nightshades, are considered generally healthy, so it might come as a bit of a surprise that these could be triggering your skin flares.

If it feels too much to completely cut out these foods from day one, simply work on reducing them. The important focus is lots of healthy, plant-based greens on your plate. You might also find you're naturally more inclined to cut out certain foods as your tastebuds begin to change. I used to love milk chocolate and always considered dark chocolate too bitter. These days, I much prefer that slightly bitter flavour and find milk chocolate too sweet.

SUGAR

So, let's start with sugar. When we ingest sugar, or other high-glycemic foods that rapidly convert to sugar, our body breaks down these carbohydrates into glucose. Simple carbs, like refined sugar, white bread, wheat pasta and fizzy drinks, cause our insulin levels to spike, which leads to a burst of inflammation throughout the body. Inflammation produces enzymes that break down collagen and elastin, resulting in sagging skin and wrinkles. Digested sugar permanently attaches to the collagen in our skin through a process known as glycation. Aside from increasing the effects of ageing, glycation can also exacerbate skin conditions like acne and rosacea.

DAIRY AND EGGS

My plan and recipes in *Radiant* were largely vegan, aside from a few eggs and occasionally honey. I personally stopped eating eggs a couple of years ago after learning more about the treatment of chickens. Up until then I'd always been fortunate enough to have a steady supply of fresh eggs from my local farm, but an early evening visit from a hungry Mr Fox put paid to that. I've since learned that eggs can be quite a problematic trigger for skin conditions, particularly for eczema. In fact, they're considered one of the most common food allergies in patients with atopic dermatitis, alongside milk and peanuts.

Dairy products, including cow's milk, yogurt, butter and cheese, are the second most common food allergy seen in eczema sufferers. They can also cause damage to the lining of the gastrointestinal tract. When the gut lining is damaged, tiny holes allow larger food particles to enter the body and allergic reactions and sensitivities can result. Naturopaths often refer to this as "leaky gut" and the term doctors

Think about all the positives this new lifestyle is going to bring to every corner of your life

use is "increased intestinal permeability". Furthermore, whey and casein are the proteins in milk that stimulate growth and hormones in calves. When humans digest these proteins, they release a hormone similar to insulin, called IGF-1, known to trigger acne breakouts.

NIGHTSHADES

For psoriasis, psoriatic arthritis and lupus sufferers, nightshades could be exacerbating flares. Nightshade vegetables include: tomatoes, white potatoes (but not sweet potatoes), peppers (but not black pepper), chillies, paprika, goji berries, aubergine (eggplant), tobacco and ashwagandha.

Typically considered healthy, these foods feature prominently in most vegetarian restaurant menus and in every vegan cookbook I own! For the majority of people, they pose no threat whatsoever and should be included as part of a healthy, plant-based diet. But for those of us with skin conditions, they can prove incredibly problematic.

Nightshade is a botanical family of more than 2,000 plant species, more technically called *Solanaceae*. The majority of them are inedible and many are highly poisonous – you might have heard of "deadly nightshade".

The reason nightshade vegetables are thought to be difficult to eat, specifically for those of us with skin diseases, is due to a type of saponin they contain called glycoalkaloids. This family of chemical compounds is believed to stimulate and exaggerate an immune system response. The nightshade family is particularly problematic for anyone struggling with an autoimmune condition such as psoriasis, arthritis or lupus.

If you notice that excluding nightshades leads to improvements in your skin, they could well be an important trigger for you. You will need to be vigilant when it comes to buying pre-packaged food, sauces and even spice blends, which can contain hidden potato starch, chilli spice and tomato. If nightshades are your trigger, they can be notoriously difficult to reintroduce. But don't worry – I've got you covered. See page 61 for my game-changing Tomato-less Sauce. It's simple, delicious, perfect for everything from bolognese to taco salsa, and nightshade-free.

A NATURAL HEALING PLAN

It's common to be tempted to think about a natural skin-healing plan in the same way we approach pharmaceutical medicine. We want a single cure and a time frame. If there was one magic food I could bottle and prescribe, alongside a time frame detailing how long it would take to kick in, I guarantee everyone would buy it! We've become so used to instant satisfaction that it's difficult to be patient these days. Natural healing is very different, and while I share your frustrations in dealing with a skin condition you want to rid yourself of, approaching it with a quick-fix attitude is only going to frustrate you. As hard as it might feel, it's important to embrace the journey.

This isn't to say you might not see amazing results over a short period of time (many people do), but rather than focus on that as a goal, I want you to really think about all the positives this new lifestyle is going to bring to every corner of your life. Thinking about the long-term implications of making these changes is really important. Coming at it with an attitude of "I'll try it for 30 days," is okay, but if you're not seeing visible changes on your skin within that month, think about the other areas of your health where you might have seen improvement. Less itching, better sleep, weight loss or gain, more energy … Trust that this way of nourishing your body is working on the inside; you just need to give it a little time to reflect on the outside.

It's important to treat all the different parts of the body as a single entity

Naturopathy is a distinct and complete system of health care which promotes the body's own self-healing mechanism. It's important to view all the different parts of our body as a single entity and treat it as a whole. The more of these healing processes you adopt, the stronger your chances of seeing results. But remember to balance that need with something that's going to be sustainable for you.

For me, the key to success was about being super strict for the first few weeks and months, and then learning to adapt my diet and incorporate new foods as I went along. I was so scared that my skin was going to flare up again that I used to suffer recurring nightmares about it. These put me off deviating from my very strict regime, but eventually I realized I had to find a balance. For you, that might be choosing certain things to work on first, or it could be that you stick to eating well during the week, but allow a bit more flexibility on the weekend.

I've designed this book so you can work at your own pace; you can incorporate the bits you're ready to change right now, and work on the rest as you go along. I want this book to feel like a toolbox you can reach into at any time. When things are difficult, remember you are in control. Empower yourself by referring back to the book and choosing something to implement, change or work on. Every positive step you take is strengthening that circle of wellbeing.

GOOD GUT HEALTH

Instead of focusing on what we see on the outside, let's concentrate on what's going on beneath the surface. We've already established that our skin relies on good gut health. The gut is our gastrointestinal tract, it's everything inside us from our mouth down to our bottom.

It's hardly a great revelation that the gastrointestinal tract is important to human health: it's responsible for transporting food from our mouth down to our stomach, for breaking it down, absorbing the nutrients from that food and filtering any waste products or toxins out. Those nutrients we absorb are the building blocks of cells, including our skin.

But in recent years, scientists have discovered that our gut has an even bigger, more complex job than previously thought. It has been linked to numerous aspects of health that have seemingly nothing to do with digestion – everything from immunity to emotional stress and chronic illness.

Our digestive tract is full of trillions of bacteria that not only help us process food, but also assist our body to maintain overall wellbeing. Research on these bacteria, often referred to as "the microbiome", is still relatively new, but studies have already found that certain environments, foods, behaviours, sleep patterns and medication can influence our gut health for better or worse.

From the moment we're born, exposure to germs and bacteria (within reason) can strengthen our gut microbiome. Spending time in nature, digging in the dirt and playing with animals are all things that can help establish a healthy gut. Modern day excessive use of antibacterial cleansing products and antibiotic medication is preventing our immune systems from strengthening as they should. Once we grow older, other factors begin coming into play.

I'm going to focus on diet, sleep, exercise,

mindfulness and what we apply to the surface of our skin: five key pillars that I believe make up the essential jigsaw pieces in gut health – and in turn your skin-healing journey. The great news is, you can start work on every single one of these right away.

CELEBRATE THE SMALL STUFF

When it comes to achieving goals, most clients come to me with one mission … to clear their skin. When we're battling chronic skin disease, much else in life can appear irrelevant. We focus intently on just that one goal – life would be perfect, if only we had clear skin. That's not true of course. But while it impacts so many different aspects of our lives – relationships, study, job opportunities, social occasions, confidence – it's easy to blame our skin for all that's not well in our world and to focus on it as our singular source of happiness.

Making dietary, fitness and lifestyle changes can feel huge. Trying to do this all at once can become almost overwhelming. My step-by-step approach to gradually strengthening your circle of wellbeing is designed to split this process into much more manageable, practical, bite-sized chunks that feel infinitely more achievable.

This might require patience, and patience is a virtue with which I most definitely struggle. If I want something, I want it now! When tackling this life-encompassing skin disease, it can be easy to get frustrated pretty quickly. The battle is exhausting and seemingly unending, so we really should spend more time celebrating the small stuff. When it comes to working toward our big goal, it can help to break that into manageable pieces. I have clients who found it impossible to go 24 hours drinking just juice. For someone who starts out struggling to complete a 24-hour juice cleanse, achieving three days feels magnificent. Similarly, I worked with a lady whose foot skin was so painful she could barely walk, so completing her first 5km local park run was like winning the New York City Marathon!

Celebrating the small stuff motivates us. It inspires others around us. It helps us establish important habits to keep going. Each peak marks a milestone and takes us one step closer to our ultimate goal. Celebrate the journey, not just your final destination.

WHAT'S HOLDING YOU BACK?

Excuses are a way of rationalizing failures. They are invented reasons we create to defend our behaviour, to postpone taking action or simply as a means of neglecting responsibility. We are all guilty of making excuses, whether it's feeling too tired, not having enough time or not knowing where to begin. Get clear on your excuses, so that next time you hear yourself rationalizing failure you become aware of it and take responsibility for your actions.

Don't ever think that a goal-setting exercise is futile. Whenever you're feeling overwhelmed, make a concerted effort to take time out to reignite your passion. Believe in yourself, connect with others on a similar journey and reach out for help when you need it. It may feel tough at times, but trust me, it's worth it.

ACCOMPLISH YOUR GOALS

Why do you want to achieve your goal?

What steps do you need to take?

What do you feel is holding you back?

How will you feel when you have achieved your goal?

What is one thing you can do today to begin working towards your goal?

How will you celebrate along the way?

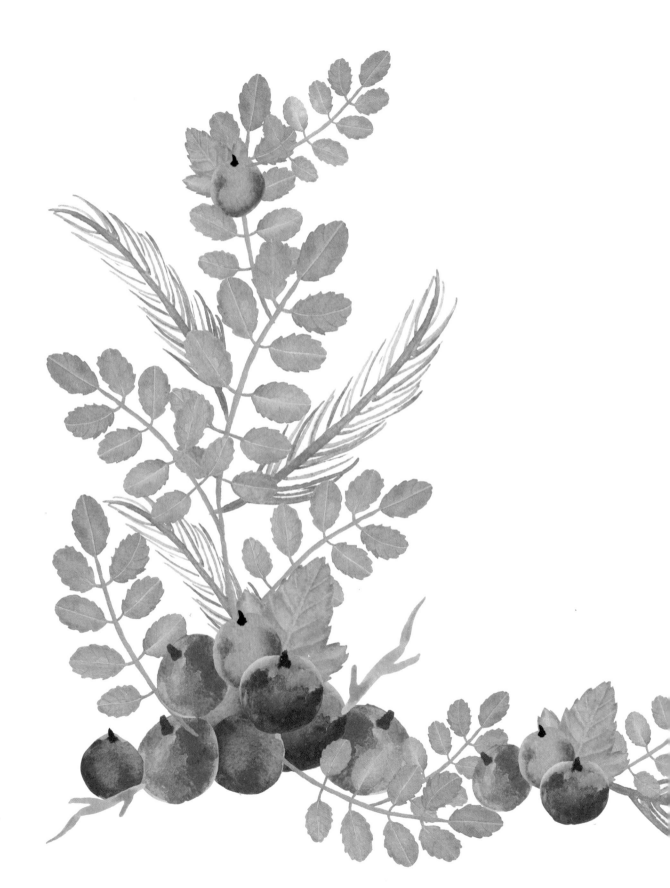

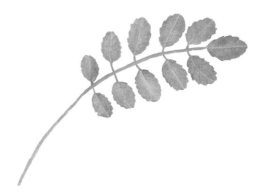

{ chapter 1 }

diet

Since we're talking about the gut – the part of our body responsible for digesting food – let's begin by considering the most obvious factor to play a role in our microbiome; what we eat. A diet low in fibre, fruit and vegetables can have a seriously negative impact on our gut health. The importance of a plant-based diet becomes clear when we acknowledge fruit and vegetables as the very best, alkaline sources of soluble fibre – essential for "feeding" the good bacteria in our gut. Other high-fibre foods include beans and pulses, such as chickpeas and lentils, brown or wholegrain rice, nuts and seeds, oats and sweet potatoes. You'll find I use plenty of these ingredients in my recipes, as incorporating a wide variety in your diet each day is vital for good gut health.

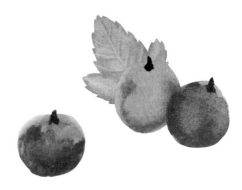

PAULA'S STORY

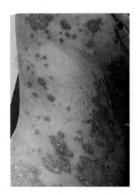 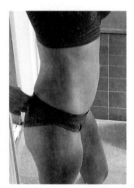

"I've battled psoriasis for more than 35 years. I was diagnosed when I was 11 years old. It appeared out of nowhere and I was absolutely covered. The patches ran across my neck and forehead, the plaques formed what looked like a map of England across my back. While my friends enjoyed their teenage years, I was so self conscious.

At one stage it got so bad that I was hospitalized. The doctors recommended daily treatment baths and covered me in steroid creams – it went on for seven weeks. My mum would find me standing in front of a mirror crying my eyes out. Nobody seemed to know how to stop this disease and it just kept getting worse.

The condition impacted my relationships and friendships. Being intimate was daunting. I never felt as though anyone would be attracted to me. I didn't feel comfortable going swimming or sunbathing.

Last February, in severe pain, I found Hanna's book, *Radiant*. Day-by-day, my skin improved. I focused on a diet full of fresh fruit, vegetables, nuts and seeds, instead of the processed foods I'd eaten before. After 17 days, my skin was clear. My life has completely changed. I wear whatever I want, I go to the gym, and I'm not a prisoner in my own skin anymore. I can't begin to describe the difference between myself a year ago and now. It's not just physical – my mindset is completely different. I'm proud of my body and I feel like a new woman."

PLANT-BASED BENEFITS

Making major dietary changes can feel quite overwhelming. Rather than focus on what you can't eat, it's really important to switch your mindset and think about what you can eat. Don't stress too much about considering everything you might need to begin excluding from your current diet; think first about all the amazing new foods you're going to enjoy.

If all you can envisage to begin with is incorporating a single green juice each morning, that's a huge step in the right direction. Increasing your water intake, adding more vegetables to your plate, swapping sweets for fresh fruit … the intention is to make simple changes step-by-step that, over the subsequent weeks and months, come to make a massive difference.

WHAT IS PLANT-BASED?

"Plant-based" is not my fancy way of saying vegan! Vegans are well catered for these days, so a vegan diet can include junk food, crisps, chocolate, cake, etc., but we don't really want to consume more of those. Plant-based is just that: a diet focused mostly on incorporating heaps of plant foods – what you do around that can be flexible.

I choose a diet free of animal products, because I believe it to be the very best way to keep inflammation low in my body. It also aligns with my ethics and love of animals. This is a personal choice, based on my own experience and healing journey over the past six years. If your diet currently includes a lot of meat, the thought of becoming vegan might be a little overwhelming. If your diet includes some meat, it may not be a big deal for you to exclude it, or you may already be vegetarian. Whatever your current stance on consuming animal products, there's no escaping the truth; lowering meat consumption is better for our health and better for the health of our planet. I like the term "plant-based" because we're simply concentrating on eating more plants and fewer animal products. Whichever stage of the transition you're at, that's your key mission.

WHY EXCLUDE ANIMAL PRODUCTS?

The World Health Organization has classified processed meats, including ham, salami and bacon, as a Group 1 carcinogen, which means that there is strong evidence these products cause cancer. Red meat, such as beef, lamb and pork, has been classified as a "probable" cause of cancer.

Our metabolism – the part of us that converts food into energy – is sometimes compared to fire. Both involve a chemical reaction that breaks down a solid mass. When things burn, an ash residue is left behind. This metabolic waste can be classed as alkaline, neutral or acidic. Our body's pH sits at around 7.4 and, just like our core body temperature, this figure is not designed to fluctuate wildly. However, in today's stressful environment with us ever reliant on convenience foods, it can be hard for our body to maintain that equilibrium. It's the reason incorporating lots of alkaline foods can take the pressure off the body and help us to redress the balance.

Meat is considered acid-forming on the pH scale, with red meat up there as one of the most acidic foods we can consume. It's difficult for the body to break down and digest, and requires extra work from the kidneys. As a result, meat consumption produces too much acidity, which in turn impacts the body's immune defences. This can not only increase the risk of skin infections, but also contributes to chronic skin disease. The average person includes meat in meals at least twice a day.

That's a huge amount of acidic, animal protein for the body to break down. In this book, we want to reduce inflammation and soothe the gut, but meat consumption contradicts what we're trying to accomplish.

The truth is, it doesn't matter how your meat was raised or produced or whether the cow bounced about in its field living a happy life. There are compounds naturally found in animal products or created during processing that increase their inflammatory profile. These things exist in all meat, regardless of organic agriculture. The overall aim, for the sake of our health and the health of our planet, is to reduce our consumption of meat and focus on plant-based meals instead.

MEAT ALTERNATIVES

The reason I don't encourage replacing meat with meat substitutes is that, unless you're excluding meat purely for ethical reasons, meat replacements are not always a suitable alternative. Highly processed soy foods are generally packaged to look like regular sausages and burgers, and while the taste has massively improved over the years, there are still healthier foods to put on your plate. Remember I'm talking about "plant-based", so if it's possible to incorporate more plants, that would be ideal. My favourite meat replacement solutions are actually much easier to make than you'd think, using a combination of mushrooms, jackfruit, buckwheat and lentils to create a delicious, filling texture that adds significant plant-based benefits.

My favourite meat replacement solutions include mushrooms, jackfruit, buckwheat and lentils

PLANT-BASED PLATE

50%   Your plate should primarily be made up of healthy vegetables and fruit

15%   Grains and complex carbs such as quinoa

15%   Vegan protein such as tofu and tempeh

10%   Legumes such as beans and lentils

5%   Nuts, seeds and healthy oils

5%   Sweet treats such as dark chocolate

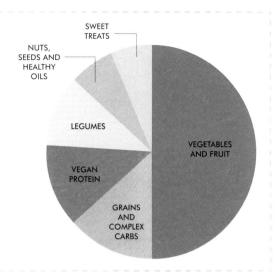

SWEET TREATS

NUTS, SEEDS AND HEALTHY OILS

LEGUMES

VEGETABLES AND FRUIT

VEGAN PROTEIN

GRAINS AND COMPLEX CARBS

SKIN-FRIENDLY PLANT-BASED PLATE

In an ideal world, this is how your plate should look at every mealtime. Now I know it's impossible to achieve that, especially at breakfast or when you're grabbing lunch on the go, but this is a great visual reminder of what you should aim for. Focus on lots of vegetables and fruit, a smaller percentage of complex grains such as quinoa or wild rice, the same amount of vegan protein sources, some legumes, a few nuts, seeds and oils, and healthy treats such as dark chocolate to take the edge off those sweet cravings.

SHOULD WE BE BUYING ORGANIC?

The moment I mention transitioning to a plant-based diet, one of the first questions I'm often asked is whether those plant foods need to be organic. The fact is, buying organic means more than better quality fruit and vegetables. Organic translates to fewer pesticides, no artificial additives, no preservatives, and in the case of animal produce, better welfare and no routine use of antibiotics. The reasons why organic food costs more are connected to the

reasons we choose organic in the first place. Weeds can't simply be sprayed away, which means farmers have more labour-intensive work. Wouldn't it be amazing if we all had the resources and budget to go 100 per cent organic forever?

I appreciate the huge benefits. I hosted a skin-healing retreat in Andalusia, Spain in 2018. We took guests to a yoga class, which was led by a wonderful couple, Jackie and Alain, who also invited us to their olive farm during harvesting season. We immediately noticed that the land on which their trees were planted was green and vibrant with thick green grasses growing beneath the olives. The farm next door didn't look like that: the soil beneath their olive trees was deep orange and barren (as you so often see across the acres of olive groves in Spain). Alain explained to us that through growing olives organically they did not use pesticides, which in turn allowed wheat grasses to grow abundantly. To olive farmers this is usually a hindrance as it catches in netting during harvest, however, Jackie and Alain's horses eat the grass and produce manure, which in turn feeds the trees. Butterflies and bees bob between flowers.

Seeing these farms side by side and witnessing the unmissable stark contrast between lush green life and dead brown soil, across a very clear dividing line, stayed with me. Not only did Jackie and Alain's olive oil taste amazing, it was also a lesson in choosing how we decide to nourish our bodies.

In everyday life, the division is not quite as stark. Often all we see on the supermarket shelves are two fairly identical looking fruits or vegetables alongside one another, with the one labelled "organic" featuring a higher price tag. If I shop at my local organic store, there is no doubt that the produce there tastes and smells infinitely better; the carrots have the same flavour as those we pulled up from the veg patch as kids, the apples taste like the ones we picked from the trees – it's like eating "real" food again, but the difference isn't just in the flavour. When we're making this conscious decision to nourish ourselves, improve gut health and, in turn, our skin, it seems logical to invest in the very best food we can afford. Although many factors can influence our gut bacteria during our lifetime, exposure to pesticides is a particularly important one. Reducing our ingestion of pesticides wherever possible can also help to limit any negative impact on that all-important gut microbiome.

With that said, shopping organic 100 per cent of the time is easier said than done. The dilemma is the same for many of us. On average, organic produce costs about 47 per cent more than conventional versions of the same foods, which are grown using synthetic pesticides and herbicides. However, price differences can vary widely. I think the key is to include some organic foods in your diet where possible, but not to stress if it's simply not an option. There are ways to make ordering organic more attainable:

- Frozen organic food is still good for you and it's often cheaper than fresh organic choices. Studies have shown that freshness can be preserved when frozen soon after harvest, and frozen foods are still filled with their nutritional benefits once thawed.
- Most big supermarket chains now have their own-brand organic ranges, which can be cheaper.
- Buying direct from the farm, picking your own or ordering a local veg box delivery can be a great option for cheaper organic produce. Organic veg box deliveries will provide a good base of ingredients for the week, save you time shopping and help support local farms. Many offer the option to exclude certain veg, so for example, if you're avoiding nightshades, you can exclude them upon placing your order.
- Grow your own. From simple window-box herbs to using small raised beds to grow greens, even the tiniest outside space can be transformed into a mini kitchen garden. Try growing a couple of container plants and gradually expanding your garden as you gain confidence. Remember to save seeds to plant next year.
- Seasonal organic produce is cheaper than out-of-season produce. Firstly because it hasn't had to be shipped halfway across the world and secondly because it is more

We're making a conscious decision to nourish ourselves and improve our gut health.

abundant. Eating seasonally is a great way to make organic affordable.

To help us strike a balance, the Environmental Working Group (EWG) releases an updated Shopper's Guide to Pesticides in Produce (aka the Dirty Dozen and Clean Fifteen) every year. If you can't afford to buy all organic, then it's worth consulting this list as a rough guide to help you choose which foods to invest in and which you needn't worry too much about. All research agrees on the health benefits of a diet that includes lots of fruit and vegetables. Eating fresh produce, whether organic or conventional, as budget allows, is essential for good health. If you want to reduce your intake of pesticides, only buying organic versions of the Dirty Dozen foods is a good place to start – a current example is below. Just don't let these lists influence you to limit your overall consumption of fresh produce.

FINE TO BUY REGULAR

Avocados	Asparagus
Sweetcorn	Kiwis
Pineapples	Cabbages
Frozen sweet peas	Cauliflower
Onions	Cantaloupes
Papayas	Broccoli
Aubergines	Mushrooms
(Eggplants)	Honeydew melons

BEST TO BUY ORGANIC

Strawberries	Peaches
Spinach	Cherries
Kale	Pears
Nectarines	Tomatoes
Apples	Celery
Grapes	Potatoes

DAIRY

Since we're talking about transitioning away from animal products, let's discuss dairy. Skin conditions are complex little beasts. Foods that massively trigger one person can have a less dramatic impact on somebody else. That said, there are certain food groups that repeatedly crop up as being a sure-fire trigger, and in the case of acne, rosacea and eczema, dairy is most certainly a culprit. So, why are dairy products such an issue?

Consider it logically. While we were endlessly sold on the benefits of milk during the eighties as essential for bone strength, we are the only species that consumes milk into adulthood. We are also the only ones to drink the milk of other animals. Biologically, cow's milk is meant to feed a rapidly growing calf. We are not calves, and as adults we no longer need to grow. In fact, around three quarters of the world's adult population is unable to break down lactose, the natural sugar present in milk – this is called lactose intolerance. After infancy, it becomes more difficult for humans to break down lactose and digest it. Your skin breakout could be due to a lactose sensitivity or allergic reaction. From an evolutionary perspective, dairy is not necessary for optimal health.

Dairy cows are sometimes treated with artificial hormones that affect their milk supply. One theory is that these hormones can interact with our own hormones, confusing our body's endocrine system and signalling breakouts. This can trigger hormone-related skin conditions, and seems to exacerbate specifically acne, rosacea and eczema. Another theory is that the growth hormones naturally present in milk aggravate certain skin conditions and when combined with the high levels of refined foods and processed sugars in our Western diet, disrupt our insulin levels and make skin more prone to acne.

DAIRY ALTERNATIVES

SOY

Soy is typically consumed whole or fermented in Asian diets, whereas in Western countries, soy is mostly processed or in supplement form. Whole soy products are the least processed foods, such as edamame, which are immature (green) soybeans. Soy milk and tofu are also made from whole soybeans. Fermented soy products are processed using traditional methods and have been cultured with beneficial bacteria, yeast or mould. These include soy sauce, tempeh and miso. Some believe that fermenting soy improves its digestibility and absorption in the body, as this process partially breaks down soy's sugar and protein molecules. Processed soy products include burgers and sausages made using soy.

Studies may seem to present conflicting conclusions about soy, but this is largely due to the wide variation in how soy is studied. In some studies, it's been shown to offer several benefits, such as improving cholesterol levels, fertility and menopause symptoms. That said, it remains controversial as weak evidence from animal studies suggests that it could be linked to breast cancer, poor thyroid function, dementia and interference with male hormones.

I limit my soy intake to tempeh, miso, tofu and occasionally edamame beans, which I'll add to a salad. Besides that, I'll usually opt for an alternative plant-based milk.

PLANT-BASED MILKS

So, if soy milk is off the menu, what's the alternative? There are lots of plant-based milks that are fantastic options. Check the ingredients; I would always recommend choosing unsweetened milk that contains no added sugars.

Almond milk – probably the most popular dairy-free option, it's incredibly versatile and inexpensive. Plus, if you're feeling really fancy, you can make it yourself.

Coconut milk – super rich and creamy and loaded with healthy fats. Canned varieties are much thicker than cartons and aren't ideal for drinking, but they're awesome for making creamy curries or vegan ice cream.

Rice milk – a great alternative if you're avoiding nuts and soy. Light and refreshing.

Oat milk – loaded with fibre, oat milk is naturally sweet, making it perfect for baked goods such as cakes and cookies. It's also a great choice for lattes. Not recommended, however, if you have a serious gluten allergy.

Hazelnut milk – naturally sweet with a strong flavour. It's one of my favourites for making muesli and using in hot chocolate.

CHEESE

There are entire recipe books dedicated to the art of vegan cheese making! While it's not impossible, it's quite involved, and let's face it, infinitely more complex than opening a packet of pre-grated Cheddar. The good news is, there are more and more vegan cheeses creeping onto our supermarket shelves. I'll often use a simple savoury cashew cream as a cheese-style pasta sauce (see the Vegan Mac 'n' Cheese on page 65), but aside from special occasions, I mostly buy ready-made vegan cheese.

ICE CREAM

Some of the biggest non-vegan ice-cream brands in the world are jumping on the plant-based ice-cream bandwagon. It's big business. Most still contain heaps of refined sugar, but healthier options are also appearing on our shelves. Vegan ice cream is actually pretty simple to make. A combination of canned coconut milk, frozen bananas and maple syrup and you're all set. Just add your favourite flavour.

BUTTER

Non-dairy margarines used to be pretty dire in terms of healthy ingredients. Recently, vegan butters have been getting better, typically made with avocado, rapeseed and sunflower oils. There are some decent options on the shelves. Many still contain emulsifiers and palm oil, so if you're stuck for options you could always make your own (see page 50).

MAKE THINGS SIMPLE

If this is the first time you've considered dietary changes in order to heal your skin, the thought of completely changing the way you prepare meals might feel a little overwhelming. We all have such busy lives these days, and while the health benefits of celery juice, fresh salads and homemade, plant-based stews are all well and good, when are we meant to find the time to conjure them up? It might also be that you simply don't enjoy cooking and rely on shop-bought ready-meals and convenience foods. My schedule is insanely busy much of the time, so I'm totally with you on this. Anything we can do to make life easier will also make it less painful to stick to a healthier regime.

FREEZE

Freezing is one of the oldest and most widely used methods of food preservation. Freezing juices and foods not only makes our lives so much simpler, it also preserves their taste, texture and nutritional value better than any other method.

There are certain foods that can become damaged through freezing, because the formation of ice crystals causes the cell membranes to break up. This has no adverse effects in terms of safety (indeed some bacterial cells would also be killed), but food can lose its crispness. Foods that do not tolerate freezing very well include things such as salad leaves, mushrooms and soft fruits. Delicate

FREEZER TIPS

- » Freezers should be kept at or below -18°C (65°F).
- » In contrast to refrigerators, your freezer should be packed as tightly as possible. This actually allows it to function better.
- » While I much prefer using glass jars in cupboards and the refrigerator, you're better freezing in food-grade silicone bottles or containers. These will help protect foods in the freezer and prevent freezer burn. Glass might also crack as liquids expand.
- » Allow hot foods to cool before placing them into the freezer, as failing to do so can raise the freezer temperature and may adversely affect other foods.
- » Ensure that frozen food is completely defrosted before cooking. Food that has been frozen and defrosted should never be refrozen.

vegetables like lettuce practically disintegrate when they're frozen and then thawed. Freezing creamy sauces can cause them to separate and "break" or curdle when defrosted. That said, most foods can be safely kept in your home freezer for 3–12 months without loss of quality.

WHAT TO FREEZE

Soups, stews and casseroles are my favourite things to freeze. There's nothing better than knowing you've got a healthy, homemade ready-meal that's good to go after a long day at work. I love to freeze my Tomato-less Sauce (see page 61) in silicone muffin trays so that I can pop out a portion when a recipe calls for it! And bulk freezing cold-pressed juices really helps me stay on track during a detox cleanse.

Frozen fruits and vegetables are great, too, and may even be healthier than some of the fresh produce sold in supermarkets. Frozen produce tends to be processed at its peak ripeness, a time when, as a general rule, vegetables are most nutrient-packed. Buying frozen greens is a great way to ensure there's always an extra vegetable you can add to casseroles and stews. Buying bags of frozen berries gives you something extra healthy to add to porridge or smoothie recipes. Plus, these are all inexpensive options.

Note: Freezing foods renders bacteria inactive but doesn't actually kill anything. That means if your food went into the freezer contaminated, once defrosted it will still harbour the same harmful bacteria. Cooking it to the recommended temperature is the only way to ensure that your food is safe.

BULK PREP

Besides looking at the way we store foods, thinking about how we prepare foods can also make sticking to a healthy plan much easier. Spending a couple of extra hours prepping when you have time to spare on a Sunday

afternoon can save you precious minutes when life takes over during the week. When we're busy navigating the roller coaster of everyday stuff, the thought of cooking all our meals from scratch can often feel incredibly overwhelming.

A lack of preparation can be the reason we reach for a ready-meal, call in at a fast food place on the way home from work or order a takeaway when we're crashed out, exhausted on the sofa. Short for "meal preparation", meal prep is the act of planning, preparing and packaging meals and snacks in advance. Keep in mind there is no right or wrong way to do meal prep, as it's all about what works for you personally. The ultimate goal is to save time in the kitchen and to have access to healthy meals during the week.

Besides saving us time, meal prep can help with portion control, ensuring we get the perfect balance of nutrients each day. It makes us think more about what we're putting into each meal. Buying in bulk and taking advantage of the freezer can save us money as well as time. By focusing on a little additional planning like this each week, you will know exactly what you need to buy, saving the pennies and reducing food waste.

There are various ways to meal prep, not all of which involve spending an entire weekend cooking dishes for the week to come. You can choose the method that works best for you.

Make-ahead meals: Full meals cooked in advance, which can be refrigerated or frozen and reheated at mealtimes. This is particularly handy for evening meals on those days when you get home late from work.

Batch cooking: Making a large batch of a specific recipe, then splitting it into individual portions to be frozen and eaten over the coming months. This works well for soups, stews and curries and means you can make a

Batch cooking makes sticking to a healthy plan much easier.

big portion without getting bored of eating the same thing night after night all week.

Individually portioned meals: Preparing fresh meals and portioning them into individually balanced grab-and-go boxes. Designed to be refrigerated and eaten over the next few days, this is particularly handy for quick and healthy work lunches.

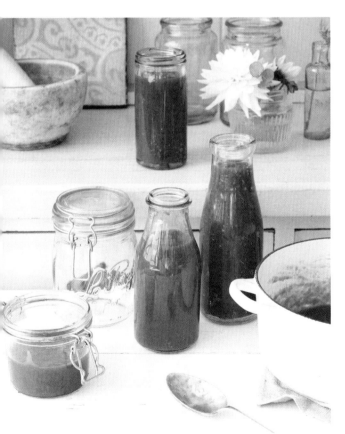

Ready-to-cook ingredients: Prepping ingredients required for specific meals ahead of time is a great way to cut down on kitchen time throughout the week. Freezing batches of Tomato-less Sauce, for example, (see page 61) can save a good hour when you want to throw together a simple spag bol.

Don't worry too much about preparing your entire week's food quota. If you wanted to bulk prep breakfast, lunch and dinner for the forthcoming work week, for example, you would need to make fifteen meals. Why not focus instead on preparing a few large batches of vegetables that can be used in various ways throughout the week, like roasted vegetables that can bulk out salads or be added to soups?

It might be worth thinking ahead to where you struggle most for time. If you find it difficult to get out of bed bright and early, prepping breakfasts might work well to set you up for the day. On the other hand, keeping batch-cooked meals in the freezer is particularly handy if you often come home late or exhausted from work.

Don't forget to label your foods. If you're freezing freshly prepared meals, you might think it's obvious to see what's inside, but once frozen, soups, stews and curries can all begin to look similar! Unless you quite like the idea of a lucky dip, a sticky label with a few simple bits of information including the preparation date can be really useful. Another advantage of a plant-based diet is that when it comes to meal prep, there simply aren't the same concerns as freezing meat or fish.

{ breakfast }

JUICING

Juicing played a huge part in my healing journey. Over the past six years I've completed many 3-, 5- and 7-day juice resets. Juicing is a fantastic way to flood the gut with a wide variety of vitamins and nutrients, while asking nothing from the body in terms of digestion.

A juicer is not the same as a smoothie maker, high-speed blender or food-processor. A juicer separates the liquid content in fruit and vegetables from the pulp, whereas a blender blitzes it altogether into a thicker smoothie. Juicing is very different. It's also important to consider that juice and smoothie recipes are not the same. A juicer recipe will not contain enough liquid to blend well. That's why smoothie recipes usually include milk or added water of some sort.

Juicing your greens can help to ensure you're getting all the vitamins you need on a regular basis. The thing I find most difficult is staying consistent. The novelty wears off, the juicer becomes a pain to clean, cold pressing greens each morning starts to feel like a chore. So, how do we make juicing an easy, enjoyable part of a long-term healing protocol?

Drinking your juice as soon as you've made it is brilliant, but bulk juicing in advance can be a huge time saver for those of us with busy lives. Being able to prep ahead of time can be the difference between sticking to a juice fast or throwing in the towel, simply because it's too time consuming to stay committed.

I would only recommend keeping juices in the fridge for a day or two max, but freezing can extend their shelf life by several months. While enzymes in fruits and vegetables can cause nutrient and quality loss during freezer storage, the potential benefits of convenience most definitely outweigh any drawbacks.

Oxidation is a reaction of nutrients in the fruit being exposed to oxygen: this is the process that causes avocados to turn brown. Juice is prone to this reaction because when fruits and vegetables are juiced, cell walls are broken down, meaning the nutrients are exposed to air, heat and light. Over time these factors will contribute to the nutrient degeneration. The longer a juice sits around, the more its nutrients will be oxidized and damaged. This is why a bright green juice can often turn a more khaki colour by lunchtime.

Freezing keeps juices safe longer, although quality begins to decline after a few months. Vitamins do degrade in the freezer, and the longer you freeze your juice, the greater the loss. For example, frozen broccoli and spinach (and the juices made with them) can lose up to 50 per cent of their vitamin C when stored for one year. But ultimately drinking juice that's been frozen is better than drinking no juice at all. To mitigate against nutrient loss and ensure juices retain their quality, pack them in airtight, heavy plastic bags or reusable plastic bottles and use them within three months. Be careful if you want to use glass bottles to store your juice as they may crack.

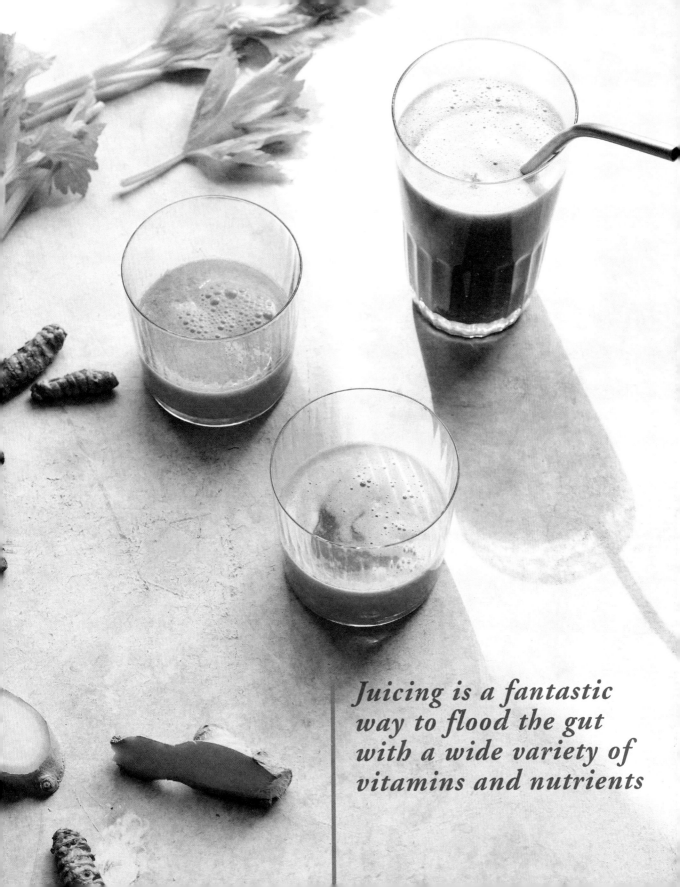

Juicing is a fantastic way to flood the gut with a wide variety of vitamins and nutrients

JUICY TIPS

- Store your juices in airtight containers.
- Freeze your juices immediately after preparation.
- Fill your container as close to the top as possible to reduce oxygen exposure (don't do this in glass as it will crack).
- Always add citrus, such as half a lemon or lime, to your juice. This will act as a natural preservative, reducing nutrient loss by boosting the vitamin C content and other antioxidants in your juice.
- Once removed from the freezer, store your juice in a dark, cool place while travelling. If you're in a warm climate, I recommend using a cooler bag with ice packs to reduce significant nutrient loss.

WHAT SHOULD WE JUICE?

My rules for juicing are simple: lots of healthy base vegetables, a stack of leafy greens, a little fruit for sweetness and lemon or lime to act as an alkalizing natural preservative. Besides this, exactly what goes through your juicer is flexible. It's good to mix things up to ensure you're getting as much variety as possible, and to benefit from lots of different vitamins and nutrients. What you juice might also depend on the fruits and vegetables available to you seasonally and locally. Here are a few of my favourite green juice recipes:

Each makes 1 juice

GREEN GODDESS
Handful of spinach
3 celery sticks
½ cucumber
2 apples
½ lemon

GLOWING GREENS
4 celery sticks
1 romaine lettuce
Handful of spring greens
¼ pineapple
½ lemon

KING OF KALE
Handful of kale
½ courgette (zucchini)
½ cucumber
3 broccoli florets
2 pears
½ lime

Wash the ingredients well. Add to the juicer, juice and enjoy.

SUPER *shots*

Super shots are a fantastic way to get a concentrated dose of juiced goodness each morning. Shots can be frozen, just like juices. They're a brilliant way to get an extra shot of nutrients into your body and offer some fantastic health benefits.

Each makes 1 shot

STREP SHOT

Strep throat is an infection commonly linked to psoriasis. Many people report a strong correlation between suffering from recurring sore throats and flares of guttate psoriasis. Prevention is always better than cure. This juice contains all the antifungal, antiviral and antibacterial ingredients you need to stop a strep flare in its tracks. I'm not going to promise it's the easiest shot to drink, but think of it as medicine!

> 1 apple
> ½ lemon
> 1 garlic clove (use fermented garlic for a softer taste, see page 101)
> 1 teaspoon apple cider vinegar

Wash the ingredients well. Peel the garlic and add to your juicer, along with the apple and lemon. Juice everything, then add the apple cider vinegar.

For powerful results, gargle the shot before drinking. If this combination feels too strong on your stomach, diluting it with water is perfectly fine.

GINGER BOOST

Ginger can help digestion, reduce nausea and fight infection. It has powerful anti-inflammatory and antioxidant effects with the power to reduce joint pain.

> 2.5cm (1 inch) piece of fresh root ginger
> 1 apple
> ½ lemon

Wash the ingredients well. Add to the juicer and drink as a shot.

TURMERIC FIRE

Turmeric is an important spice when it comes to healing inflammatory skin conditions. Not only is it anti-inflammatory, it's also a natural antiseptic and helps to keep bacteria from spreading.

> 5cm (2 inch) piece of fresh turmeric
> ½ lemon
> 1 apple
> Twist of black pepper

Wash the ingredients well. Add the turmeric, lemon and apple to the juicer. Finish with a twist of black pepper. Drink as a shot.

SMOOTHIES

Smoothies are a great alternative to juicing. Blending a smoothie involves the whole fruit or vegetable, so they are more filling. It's also easier to wash up the machine after blending.

The raw ingredients used to make a smoothie can also be prepped ahead of time and popped into freezer packs, so you can keep them ready to grab and blend when you need them. All you need to do is add your milk of choice (I like unsweetened almond or coconut milk), and blend. Even better, in the time it takes to make one smoothie from scratch, you could have an entire week's worth of smoothie packs prepped and waiting in the freezer.

Liquid: Use 100ml (3½fl oz) of plant-based milk per serving.

Produce: With fruit smoothies, you'll need a fruit base. Bananas and avocados make great bases for smoothies and don't overpower the flavour. Other ingredients that work well include: berries, mango, pineapple, peaches, spinach and kale.

Thickeners: I like my smoothies to be thick. In order to add a thick, creamy texture to your smoothies, you can include fillings that are nutritious, such as nut butters, chia seeds, flaxseeds, rolled oats or coconut yogurt.

Flavours: You might also like to give your smoothie a flavour boost by using spices, such as cinnamon or mint, or by using natural sweeteners, such as dates or maple syrup.

Boosts: This is where you can incorporate healthy add-ins and nutritional boosts that offer an extra dose of vitamins, antioxidants and even a little texture to your smoothie. Great options include flaxseeds, chia seeds, protein powder, cashews, matcha, cacao or spirulina.

One of the absolute best things about make-ahead fruit smoothie freezer bags is that you can freeze fresh produce that's about to go out of date and enjoy it later. Instead of letting bags of spinach and kale wilt beyond use, you can add them to your freezer bags and have them ready to blend any time you like. Freezing greens (besides very watery veg such as lettuce) doesn't have any impact on their flavour or texture when used in this way. Here are some tips for making smoothie packs:

- Use a freezer ziplock bag (or a freezer-safe silicone container) to make individual portions.
- Cut all produce into small pieces to make it easier to blend when frozen.
- Label the freezer bag so you know exactly which smoothie recipe you've prepared.
- Use a combination of fresh or frozen fruit.
- Add protein powder or spices when blending to incorporate more flavour or protein.

For these smoothie packs, you can simply take the frozen contents of each pack and add them to a blender, along with the milk of your choice and any other liquid ingredients like plant-based yogurt, almond butter or maple syrup. Then simply blend everything together and you're all set!

Serves 1

BLUEBERRY MUFFIN

200g (7oz) blueberries, washed and
   frozen
1 banana, chopped and frozen
100ml (3½fl oz) plant-based milk
Handful of oats

Blend everything together.

RASPBERRY CHEESECAKE

200g (7oz) raspberries, washed and
   frozen
1 banana, chopped and frozen
75ml (2½fl oz) plant-based milk
75g (2½oz) coconut yogurt

Blend everything together.

PEACH MELBA

2 peaches, chopped and frozen
1 banana, chopped and frozen
100ml (3½fl oz) plant-based milk
Handful of raspberries

Blend everything together.

SPICED PEAR

1 pear, washed, chopped and frozen
1 banana, chopped and frozen
100ml (3½fl oz) plant-based milk
½ teaspoon ground allspice
Handful of oats

Blend everything together.

MANGO MISCHIEF

200g (7oz) mango, peeled, washed,
   chopped and frozen
1 banana, chopped and frozen
100ml (3½fl oz) plant-based milk
½ teaspoon ground turmeric

Blend everything together.

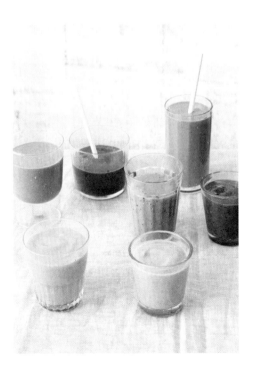

OVERNIGHT *oats*

Just like smoothies, overnight oats make a fantastic, fast, pre-made, grab-and-go breakfast. There's no cooking involved; it's literally a case of mixing all the ingredients in a glass jar and popping it in the refrigerator overnight. In the morning, you'll have a pudding-like porridge that's perfect to eat in a hurry or pop in your bag and take to work if you're really pushed for time.

Overnight oats don't have the same texture as stove-top porridge. They're creamier, denser and, in my opinion, so much tastier. To start, I'm going to talk you through my "base" recipe. Then I'll share some of my favourite add-ins, so that you can have a different variation for each day of your working week!

Oats: This is really the only ingredient that's non-negotiable. Ensure you use plain old-fashioned rolled oats and not quick oats because the consistency is best with rolled oats. Quick-cook oats can get too soggy when soaked with milk. And do not use steel cut oats because they won't soften enough without cooking. You can also use gluten-free oats if you're particularly sensitive to gluten.

Milk: You can use any plant-based milk you like: almond milk, coconut milk, cashew milk or oat milk.

Vegan yogurt: This gives the oats a tangy flavour, creamy texture and boost of protein.

Chia seeds: These seeds are packed with tons of nutrition, and they help give the oats a pudding-like texture, so I always like to include them in my base recipe.

Vanilla extract (optional): This enhances all the flavours that go into the overnight oats and is a great option if you'd prefer not to use an additional sweetener.

Sweetener (optional): I use maple syrup to sweeten the mixture, especially because oats can be a little bit bland on their own.

Mixers: This is where you can have some fun with fresh fruit, nut butters, nuts, seeds and spices. There are so many topping ideas and combinations; try some of my suggestions or experiment with your own to keep this versatile breakfast interesting.

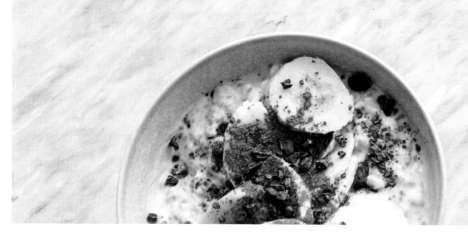

BASE RECIPE
Serves 1

50g (1¾oz) rolled oats
120ml (4fl oz) plant-based milk
60g (2oz) plant-based yogurt
1 tablespoon chia seeds
¼ teaspoon vanilla extract (optional)
1 tablespoon maple syrup (optional)
Pinch of pink Himalayan salt

Mix all the ingredients in a glass jar and pop it in the refrigerator overnight.

MIXERS

ABJ: ALMOND BUTTER JELLY
2 teaspoons almond butter
2 teaspoons sugar-free jam (or chia seed jam)

RAW CARROT CAKE
1 small carrot, grated
½ teaspoon ground cinnamon
30g (1oz) raisins
30g (1oz) walnuts

TIPS
• Make your oats in a jar with a lid for a breakfast you can grab on the go.
• Although overnight oats are typically served cold, just stir them over a gentle heat to warm through — perfect for winter mornings.
• Prep for the week. Because overnight oats usually stay good in the fridge for up to 5 days, make a batch on Sunday and have breakfast ready to go for your entire week. Just add the fruit when you're ready to eat.

BANANA CHOC CHIP
1 banana, chopped
1 tablespoon raw cacao nibs
1 tablespoon cacao powder

TROPICAL
2 tablespoons coconut flakes
75g (2¾oz) chopped pineapple
½ mango, chopped

APPLE PIE
1 small apple, deseeded and chopped
½ teaspoon ground cinnamon
30g (1oz) pecans

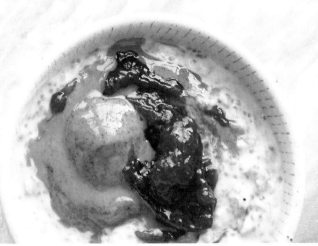
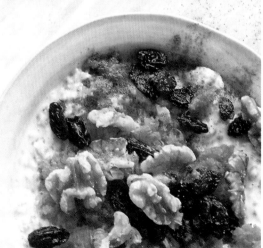

GRANOLA

Granola is such a delicious recipe to make, not just because it tastes amazing, but because it makes the entire house smell divine when it's baking! Shop-bought brands often contain lots of refined sugar. Making your own granola means you have complete control over exactly what's going into it.

HAZELNUT & CRANBERRY GRANOLA
Makes 8–10 servings

100g (3½oz) rolled oats
100g (3½oz) blanched hazelnuts, very
    coarsely chopped
50g (1¾oz) flaked almonds
50g (1¾oz) sunflower seeds
50g (1¾oz) coconut flakes
50ml (1¾fl oz) maple syrup
50ml (1¾fl oz) coconut oil, melted
½ teaspoon salt
50g (1¾oz) dried cranberries

Preheat the oven to 160°C/325°F/gas mark 3. Line a rimmed baking tray with greaseproof paper.

Toss the oats, hazelnuts, flaked almonds, sunflower seeds, coconut, maple syrup, coconut oil and salt in a large bowl.

Spread out on the baking tray and bake, tossing occasionally, until crisp and golden brown, about 20–25 minutes.

Let it cool, then stir in the cranberries. Store in an airtight container.

VANILLA COCONUT GRANOLA
Makes 8–10 servings

100g (3½oz) rolled oats
50g (1¾oz) walnuts
50g (1¾oz) flaked almonds
50ml (1¾fl oz) maple syrup
50g (1¾oz) coconut flakes
1 teaspoon ground cinnamon
Pinch of ground nutmeg
½ teaspoon salt
50ml (1¾fl oz) coconut oil, melted
2 teaspoons vanilla extract

Preheat the oven to 160°C/325°F/gas mark 3. Line a rimmed baking tray with greaseproof paper.

Toss all the ingredients together in a large bowl.

Spread out on the baking tray and bake, tossing occasionally, until crisp and golden brown, about 20–25 minutes.

Let it cool and store in an airtight container.

WARM *porridge*

If you prefer your oats warm in winter, here are a couple of my favourite cold-weather recipes. You can prep them in advance and have them ready to warm in the morning.

PERSIMMON PORRIDGE
Serves 2

100g (3½oz) porridge oats
300ml (10fl oz) plant-based milk
1 teaspoon maple syrup, plus extra to sweeten
2 teaspoons coconut oil
1 persimmon, sliced
1 peach, sliced
Ground allspice
Handful of pecans
Flaked almonds, to serve
Salt

Add the oats to a pan, stir in the plant-based milk and gently warm over a low heat for 5 minutes. Add a pinch of salt and drop of maple syrup to sweeten. Warm for a further 5 minutes over a low heat.

Meanwhile, warm the coconut oil in a pan over a low heat, add the slices of persimmon and peach, 1 teaspoon of maple syrup and a sprinkle of ground allspice. Warm and allow to bubble for 1 minute, turning the fruit over to brown evenly. Add the pecans and turn off the heat.

Serve the porridge in a bowl, topped with the fruit and sprinkled with flaked almonds and a little more ground allspice.

APPLE CRUMBLE WINTER WARMER
Serves 2

100g (3½oz) porridge oats
300ml (10fl oz) plant-based milk
1 tablespoon coconut oil
1 Bramley apple, cored and chopped
Handful of frozen berries
Pinch of ground cinnamon
Pinch of ground cloves
1 teaspoon coconut sugar or maple syrup (optional, if you like it sweet)
Pumpkin, sunflower and chia seeds
Coconut flakes
Salt

Add the oats to a pan, stir in the plant-based milk and gently warm over a low heat for 5 minutes. Add a pinch of salt. Warm for a further 5 minutes over a low heat.

In a frying pan over a low heat, gently melt the coconut oil. Add the chopped apple and frozen berries and warm slowly for 5–7 minutes. Add a pinch of cinnamon and ground cloves.

Once the porridge is ready, serve in a bowl, stirring in the cooked apples and coconut sugar (if using). Top with seeds and coconut flakes, and an extra sprinkle of cinnamon and cloves.

CHIA SEED
puddings

Chia seeds have become hugely popular over the past few years. They've actually been a staple food in Mexico for centuries. Chia seeds offer a rich vegan source of omega-3 fatty acids, antioxidants and bone-building minerals. In fact, they're so abundant in healthy fats that the word "chia" comes from the Nahautl word "chian", meaning "oily". Chia seeds are also intensely anti-inflammatory, calming and antioxidant-rich; they can provide 20 per cent of our recommended daily calcium intake and they can help us to fight ageing, soothe inflammation, reduce acne scars and keep skin radiant and healthy.

Just like overnight oats, chia pudding can be made in advance and stored in the refrigerator overnight, making it another perfect breakfast option.

CHIA SEED PUDDING
Serves 1

4 tablespoons chia seeds
200ml (7fl oz) plant-based milk
1 teaspoon maple syrup
Pinch of pink Himalayan salt

To make your chia seed pudding, add the chia seeds to the milk. Add the maple syrup and salt and stir together well. Let it set for 10 minutes, then stir again to ensure the chia seeds absorb the milk evenly.

Spoon the chia seed mixture over your chosen fruit base (see opposite) before it thickens and allow to fully set in the refrigerator overnight.

CARAMEL BANOFFEE

1 tablespoon almond butter
1 teaspoon maple syrup
Pinch of salt
1 small banana, chopped
1 quantity Chia Seed Pudding
Chopped almonds, to serve

Blend the almond butter, maple syrup and salt to create a sauce. Put the banana in the bottom of a glass jar. Pour the chia mixture over and drizzle with the sauce. Let it set overnight, then serve topped with almonds.

APPLE CRUMBLE

½ apple, cored and chopped
½ pear, cored and chopped
1 quantity Chia Seed Pudding
½ teaspoon ground cinnamon
75g (2¾oz) homemade granola (page 34)
Pecans, to decorate

Add the apple and pear to a glass jar. Stir the ground cinnamon into the chia pudding and pour on top of the fruit. Let it set overnight and serve topped with granola and pecans.

TROPICAL

1 kiwi, peeled and chopped
1 quantity Chia Seed Pudding
½ mango, deseeded
1 teaspoon coconut yogurt
Coconut flakes, to decorate

Add the kiwi to a glass jar. Pour the chia pudding on top. In a blender, purée the mango and coconut yogurt, then pour on top of the chia pudding. Let it set overnight and serve topped with coconut flakes.

RHUBARB & TURMERIC CUSTARD

2 rhubarb stalks, chopped
½ apple, cored and chopped
Maple syrup (optional)
1 quantity Chia Seed Pudding
½ teaspoon ground turmeric
75g (2¾oz) homemade granola (page 34)

Warm the chopped rhubarb and apple in a pan over a low heat for 5–7 minutes to soften (add a little maple syrup, if using, to sweeten). Spoon into a glass jar.

Stir the ground turmeric into the chia pudding and pour on top of the rhubarb. Let it set overnight and serve topped with granola.

CHERRY PIE

75g (2¾oz) frozen cherries
1 quantity Chia Seed Pudding
1 teaspoon raw cacao powder, plus extra for decorating

Warm the frozen cherries in a pan over a low heat for 5–7 minutes to defrost, then spoon into a glass jar, reserving a few for the top.

Stir the raw cacao powder into the chia seed mixture and pour the chia mixture over the cherries. Let it set overnight and serve topped with extra cherries and cacao powder.

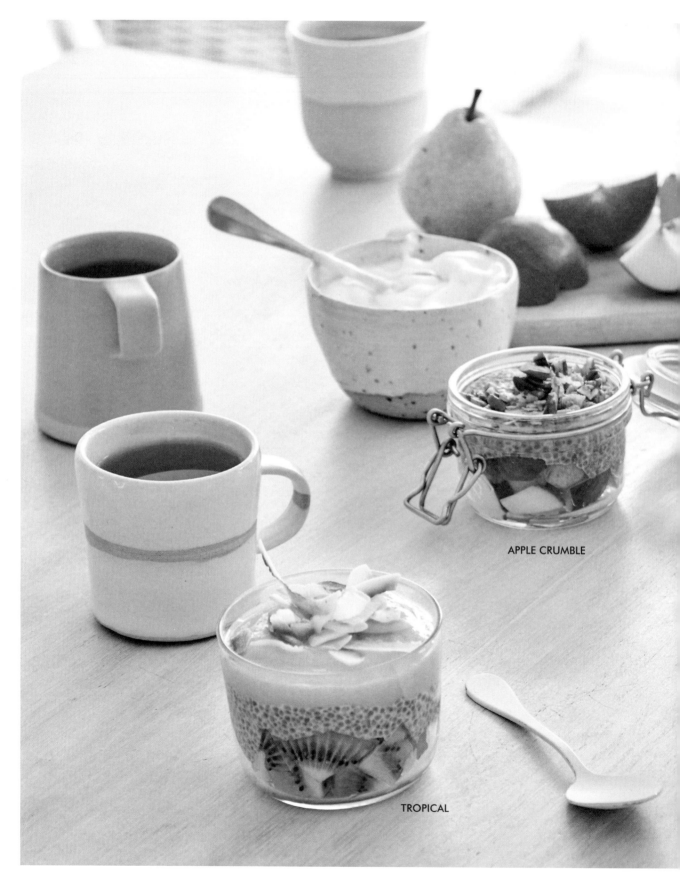

APPLE CRUMBLE

TROPICAL

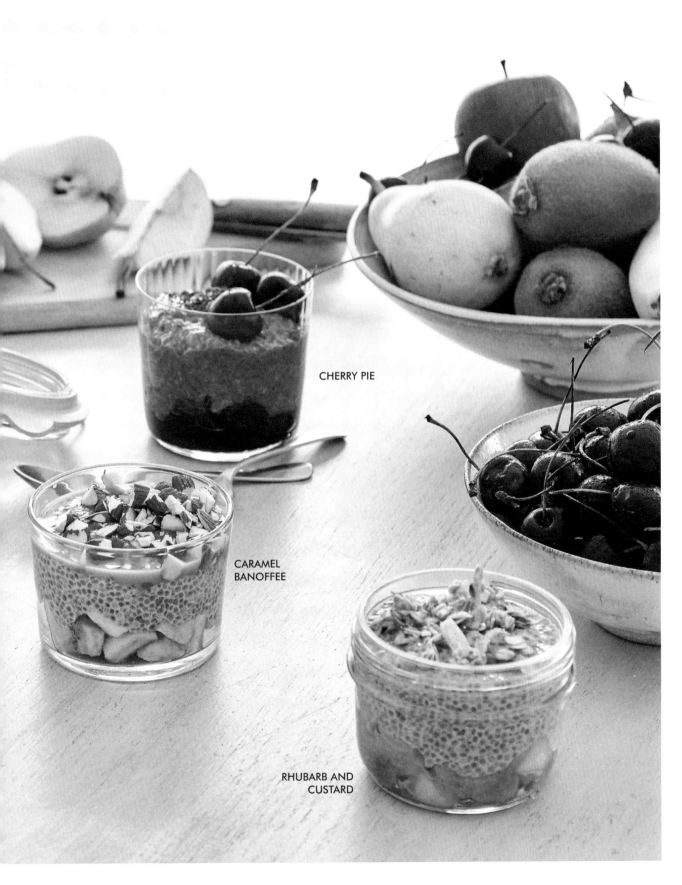

CHERRY PIE

CARAMEL
BANOFFEE

RHUBARB AND
CUSTARD

SMOKY BBQ
beans on toast

It's sometimes the simple things you miss the most. Beans on toast is a typically British breakfast. Rumour has it, Britain's biggest manufacturer of baked beans invented the dish as a marketing ploy back in 1927. It became a brilliantly inexpensive form of protein during World War II, gained notoriety that way and has become a bit of a British breakfast staple ever since.

Canned baked beans contain tomatoes, and if you're excluding nightshades (see page 11) from your diet, my tomato-less sauce is the perfect way to make this meal.

Serves 2

150ml (5fl oz) Tomato-less Sauce (see page 61)
½ teaspoon ground cumin
2 tablespoons tamari sauce
1 tablespoon coconut sugar or maple syrup
1 teaspoon English mustard
5 drops of liquid hickory smoke
400g (14oz) can haricot beans, drained

Warm the tomato-less sauce in a saucepan over a medium heat.

Add the cumin, tamari, coconut sugar or maple syrup, mustard and hickory smoke and stir well. Stir the beans through the sauce, gently warming for 5–7 minutes.

Serve on buttered bread (see the recipe for Vegan Butter on page 50).

Beans are a brilliantly inexpensive form of protein

TOFU *scramble*

I used to include eggs in my recipes quite regularly, up until my neighbour's chickens got snaffled one night by Mr Fox. Reluctant to buy even free-range brands at the supermarket, and with eggs coming up as a common intolerance for many people struggling with eczema, I began to experiment with egg alternatives.

Packed with protein, enjoying the added skin-healing benefits of turmeric and tasting completely delicious, this tofu scramble fast became a popular weekend brunch.

Serves 1

1 tablespoon Vegan Butter (see page 50)
200g (7oz) firm tofu, cubed
2 teaspoons ground turmeric
1 tablespoon nutritional yeast
1 teaspoon Dijon mustard
50ml (1¾fl oz) almond milk
Salad cress
Fresh chives, chopped
Black pepper

Melt the vegan butter in a frying pan over a low heat.

Put the tofu cubes in a bowl and use the back of a fork to mash them into scramble. Add the turmeric, nutritional yeast and mustard to the bowl and stir in the almond milk.

Add the scramble mixture to the pan and warm gently for 6–8 minutes, stirring well.

Serve with fresh cress, chopped chives and black pepper.

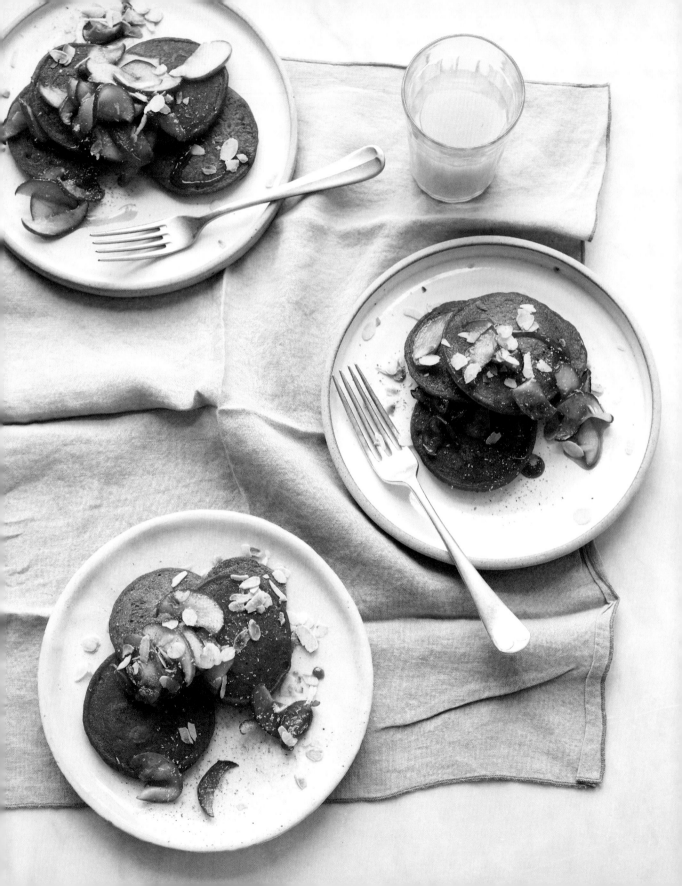

BEETROOT APPLE
pancakes

My basic pancake recipe is super simple. A quick combination of flour, milk and baking powder creates the fastest and fluffiest vegan pancakes ever!

For something a little fancier, add skin-brightening beetroot. Beets taste pretty earthy and that's why they work so well with lighter, fresher flavours such as apple, ginger and lemon.

Serves 4

1 raw beetroot
3 apples
Small piece of fresh root ginger
165g (5¾oz) self-raising flour (I use gluten-free)
100ml (3½fl oz) plant-based milk (I use almond)
1 teaspoon baking powder
2 tablespoons coconut oil, for frying
2 tablespoons maple syrup
Handful of flaked almonds
Squeeze of lemon
Fresh nutmeg, for grating
Pinch of salt

Juice the beetroot, one of the apples and the ginger. Add 125ml (4fl oz) of the resulting juice to a blender cup along with the flour, milk, baking powder and salt. Blend the ingredients together to form a smooth batter.

Add the coconut oil to a frying pan and gently heat. Carefully pour a little batter into the pan and fry for a minute or two before flipping the pancake. Stack and repeat until all the batter is used.

Thinly slice the remaining two apples and add those to the warm pan. Drizzle with maple syrup and fry for a couple of minutes to caramelize.

Stack the pancakes layered with apples. Decorate with flaked almonds, a squeeze of lemon and freshly grated nutmeg.

SAVOURY SPINACH
breakfast muffins

Are you a savoury or a sweet person at breakfast? I'm often torn between the two! If you don't fancy anything particularly sweet, these are a brilliant grab-and-go option. The beauty of breakfast muffins is making them in advance, as they store well in a tin for 3 or 4 days. Extra useful when you're rushing out of the door.

Makes 6

300g (10½oz) self-raising flour (I use gluten-free)
1 teaspoon baking powder
1 tablespoon herbes de Provence
Pinch of nutmeg
3 tablespoons nutritional yeast
4 tablespoons olive oil
350ml (12fl oz) plant-based milk (I use almond)
1 small red onion, finely chopped
Large handful of spinach
5 mushrooms, finely chopped
Pink Himalayan salt
Black pepper

Preheat the oven to 180°C/350°F/gas mark 4.

Add the self-raising flour, baking powder, herbs, nutmeg, nutritional yeast and 3 tablespoons of the olive oil to a bowl. Season with salt and pour in the milk. Use an electric whisk to combine everything well.

Add the remaining tablespoon of olive oil to a pan over a low heat. Fry the onion for 5 minutes, add the spinach and mushrooms and cook for a further 5 minutes, then stir them into the mixing bowl.

Divide the batter evenly between six silicone tray muffin cups. Sprinkle over some pepper and bake for 25 minutes.

Check the muffins are cooked using a skewer. If it comes out clean, they're done.

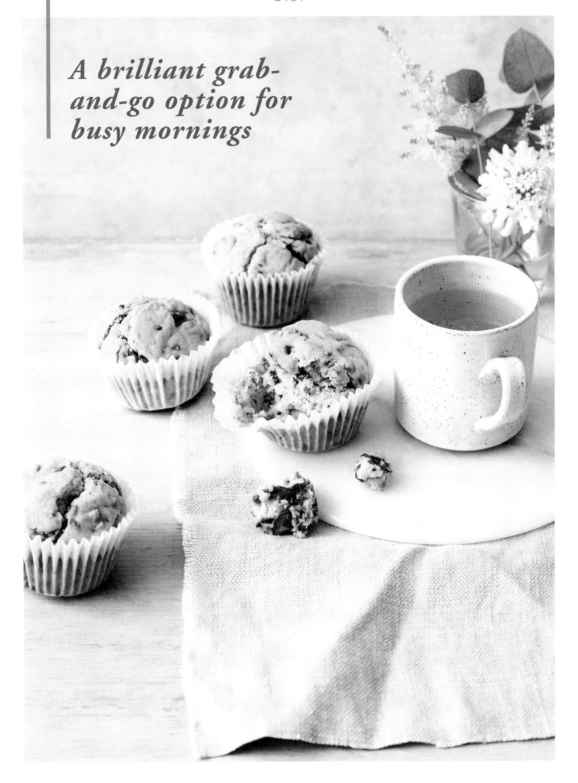

A brilliant grab-and-go option for busy mornings

SWEET POTATO
sausage hash

This tasty dish is a good excuse to bake something warm for a healthy winter brunch. It's also a fantastic way to use up any Sunday dinner leftovers, which can easily be added to the recipe.

Serves 4

2 large sweet potatoes, peeled and cubed
2 tablespoons coconut oil
6 vegan sausages
1 onion, finely chopped
2 garlic cloves, crushed
2 teaspoons ground cumin
1 teaspoon ground coriander
200ml (7fl oz) Tomato-less Sauce (see page 61)
Juice of ½ lime
Salt and black pepper
Fresh coriander (cilantro), chopped

Boil a pan of water and add the sweet potato. Cook for 5 minutes, or until almost tender. Drain and set aside.

Warm the oil in a heavy-based frying pan and cook the sausages for 8–10 minutes, turning frequently. Remove from the pan and set aside.

Return the pan to the heat and add the onions. Cook over a low heat for 8–10 minutes, or until softened.

Slice the sausages and return them to the pan, along with the sweet potatoes, garlic and spices. Pour over the tomato-less sauce and warm gently for 5–10 minutes, stirring occasionally.

Squeeze over the lime juice, season with salt and pepper to taste, and serve with fresh coriander (cilantro).

PORTOBELLO
stuffed 'shrooms

My favourite time to make these is on a lazy Sunday morning. Mushrooms are a brilliant vegan protein source and super beneficial for our skin. They contain antioxidants as well as compounds that have anti-inflammatory properties, which promote healing and fight inflammation.

Serves 4

4 large portobello mushrooms
2 tablespoons olive oil, plus more for coating the mushrooms
1 large red onion, diced
2 medium courgettes (zucchini), diced
2 garlic cloves, minced
Large handful of spinach
Pinch of dried oregano
4 tablespoons ground almonds
4 tablespoons nutritional yeast
100g (3½oz) vegan cheese, grated
Salt and black pepper

Preheat the oven to 180°C/350°F/gas mark 4. Line a baking tray with greaseproof paper.

Using a small spoon, gently remove the stalk and scoop the gills out of the inside of each mushroom. Rub the mushrooms with a bit of olive oil and place them on the baking tray, stalk side up.

Heat the oil in a pan over a low heat. Sauté the onion for 5 minutes, then add the courgette (zucchini) and garlic and warm for a further 3–5 minutes, or until softened.

Finally add the spinach, wait for it to wilt, then add the oregano, almonds and nutritional yeast. Season with salt and pepper to taste. Divide into four and stuff the mixture into each mushroom. Bake in the oven for about 30 minutes.

Add grated vegan cheese on top and then bake for a final 5–10 minutes, or until melted.

SUMMER RAINBOW
smoothie bowl

*These pretty bowls are a brilliant breakfast option in warm weather.
I love the beautiful colours and combination of textures from fresh
fruit, sprinkled nuts and seeds.*

*Keep bags of frozen mixed berries on hand in the freezer to give
you an instant vibrant base for seasonal fruits.*

Serves 1

200g (7oz) frozen berries
50ml (1¾fl oz) plant-based milk (I use almond)

TO DECORATE
Fresh raspberries, sliced
Fresh blackberries, sliced
Kiwi, peeled and sliced
1 banana, peeled and sliced
50g (1¾oz) nuts
1 tablespoon sunflower seeds
1 tablespoon coconut flakes
Edible dried or fresh flowers (optional)

Blitz the frozen berries and almond milk together and pour into a
breakfast bowl.

Decorate with sliced fresh fruit, nuts, seeds and coconut flakes. You
can even add edible dried or fresh flowers on top.

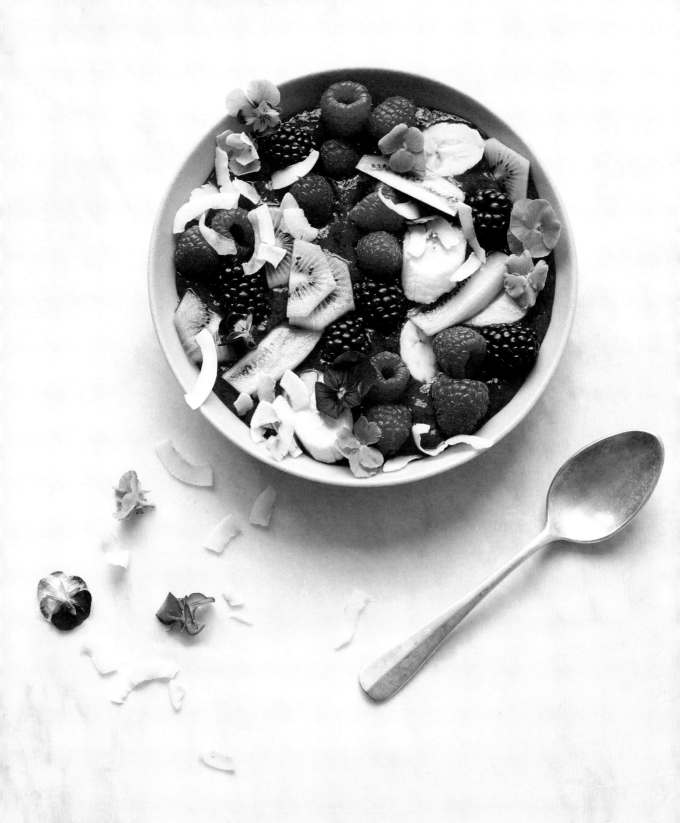

VEGAN *butter*

It's funny the foods people ask you about when you transition to a vegan diet. "What do you put on toast?" is such a common question when I explain I don't eat dairy. Jam, avocado, beans ... the same as everyone else, I guess, but without the butter. It wasn't until I made this delicious vegan butter that I realized just how much I had missed the stuff. Perfect for smothering on hot toast, but equally useful in baking, this recipe is a dairy-free game-changer.

Makes 1 block

250ml (8½fl oz) odourless or flavourless coconut oil
2 tablespoons olive oil (extra virgin tastes stronger)
100ml (3½fl oz) almond milk
1 teaspoon apple cider vinegar
2 teaspoons nutritional yeast
½ teaspoon salt
Pinch of ground turmeric

Mix the coconut oil and olive oil together using a hand whisk. In a separate bowl, whisk the almond milk and apple cider vinegar together – it should curdle!

Add the milk mixture to the oil. Add the nutritional yeast, salt and turmeric and whisk again. Pour into a butter dish and place in the fridge for 2–3 hours to firmly set. You might need to whisk once an hour as the butter sets to prevent it separating.

Remove from the fridge to soften slightly before spreading on fresh bread. This should keep in the fridge for 3–4 weeks.

TIP

If you like your toast with savoury toppings, you might enjoy a strong-tasting extra virgin olive oil, but if you want to use this butter in baking, opt for a light olive oil instead.

COURGETTE *loaf*

You might read the list of naturally sweet ingredients below and wonder what on earth courgette is doing in there. In fact, you'll barely taste the courgette at all, and it's a wonderful way to make this loaf perfectly moist. Full of vitamins A, C and K, it's also one of the easiest vegetables to grow yourself at home – and what better way to use it?

Makes 1 loaf

250g (8¾oz) self-raising flour
    (I use gluten-free)
2 teaspoons baking powder
100g (3½oz) coconut sugar
½ teaspoon salt
1 teaspoon ground cinnamon
½ teaspoon nutmeg
Pinch of ground cardamom
1 courgette (zucchini), grated
1 banana, mashed
60ml (2fl oz) coconut oil, melted
60ml (2fl oz) plant-based milk (I use
    almond)
1 teaspoon vanilla extract
Handful of walnuts, chopped

Preheat the oven to 180°C/350°F/gas mark 4.

Sift the flour into a mixing bowl and add the baking powder, coconut sugar, salt and spices. Mix together well.

Add the grated courgette (zucchini), mashed banana, coconut oil, almond milk and vanilla extract – stir to combine. It might feel as though there are not enough wet ingredients, but don't worry. Leave the mixture to stand for a couple of minutes.

Meanwhile line a 500g (1lb) loaf tin with greaseproof paper so that the paper hangs over the edge; this makes it easy to lift your loaf out once it's baked.

Return to your mixing bowl and the courgette (zucchini) will have released more water into the mix, so you should be able to form it into a thick batter. Finally, stir in the walnuts. Transfer to the lined loaf pan and smooth down evenly. Bake for 1 hour, or until a skewer inserted into the centre comes out clean.

Lift the bread out of the loaf tin using the greaseproof paper and place on to a wire cooling rack to cool before slicing.

BANANA *bread*

My lovely friend and neighbour, Sarah, is the Banana Bread Queen. Seriously, I actively let my bananas over-ripen so I can drop them in and request a loaf! The potassium in bananas is considered beneficial for fatigue, low blood sugar, cramps, brain function, bone density, kidney disorders, nerve reflexes, anxiety and stress. What better excuse do you need for a relaxing cup of sleepy night time tea and a stress-reducing slice of banana bread before bed?

Makes 1 loaf

3 medium over-ripe bananas
50g (1¾oz) coconut sugar, plus extra for sprinkling
60ml (2fl oz) coconut oil, melted
2 teaspoons vanilla extract
300g (10½oz) plain flour (I use gluten-free)
1 teaspoon bicarbonate of soda (baking soda)
1 teaspoon ground cinnamon
½ teaspoon salt
100g (3½oz) chopped pecans

Preheat the oven to 160°C/325°F/gas mark 3. Line a 500g (1lb) loaf tin with greaseproof paper.

Peel the bananas and place them into a large mixing bowl. Mash them well with the back of a fork. Add the coconut sugar, coconut oil and vanilla to the bowl. Stir until well mixed.

Add the flour to the bowl, then sprinkle the bicarbonate of soda (baking soda), cinnamon and salt on top of the flour. Stir everything together until just mixed, but don't overmix. The batter will be thick. Fold in the pecans.

Spoon the batter into the prepared loaf tin and smooth out the top with the back of a spoon. Sprinkle the top with coconut sugar.

Bake for 50 minutes, or until a skewer inserted into the centre comes out clean. Remove the tin from the oven and transfer it to a cooling rack. Allow the loaf to cool for at least 15 minutes before removing it from the tin. Slice and serve.

SUPER SEED *bread*

Nuts and seeds are great sources of skin-boosting nutrients such as vitamin E, selenium and zinc. This loaf is packed with a wonderful variety, designed to nourish and protect skin cells. Deep, dark and intense, like a wholesome German rye, with a beautifully rich, hearty, nutty flavour. I just love this bread sliced, toasted and loaded with mashed avocado.

Makes 1 loaf

75g (2¾oz) rolled oats
1 teaspoon baking powder
35g (1¼oz) sesame seeds, plus extra for decorating
40g (1½oz) flaxseeds, plus extra for decorating
40g (1½oz) chopped almonds
50g (1¾oz) sunflower seeds, plus extra for decorating
75g (2¾oz) buckwheat flour
50g (1¾oz) chia seeds, plus extra for decorating
3 tablespoons psyllium husk powder
1 teaspoon salt
50g (1¾oz) coconut oil, melted
1 tablespoon maple syrup

Preheat the oven to 150°C/300°F/gas mark 2 and line a 500g (1lb) loaf tin with greaseproof paper.

Mix all the dry ingredients in a large mixing bowl. Set aside.

In a small mixing bowl combine all the wet ingredients with 350ml (12fl oz) water. Stir the wet ingredients into the dry ones and combine. Let the batter rest for about 30–60 minutes so that the chia and flaxseeds have a chance to activate in the added moisture.

Pour the batter into the prepared baking tin and decorate the top with extra seeds before putting the bread in the oven. Bake for about 60 minutes, or until a skewer inserted into the centre comes out clean. Let the bread cool down completely before cutting into it with a serrated knife.

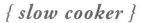

{ slow cooker }

I finally used a slow cooker for the first time last year; it's fair to say I'm a bit late to the Crockpot party! If you haven't used one before, these things are brilliant. Slow cookers are inexpensive to buy, economical to use, and fantastic for making the most of budget ingredients. They offer a healthier, low-fat method of cooking and require a minimum amount of effort. Throw everything in before you leave for work, and you'll have a delicious, nutritious meal waiting for you when you get back. They're also great for bulk cooking and freezing.

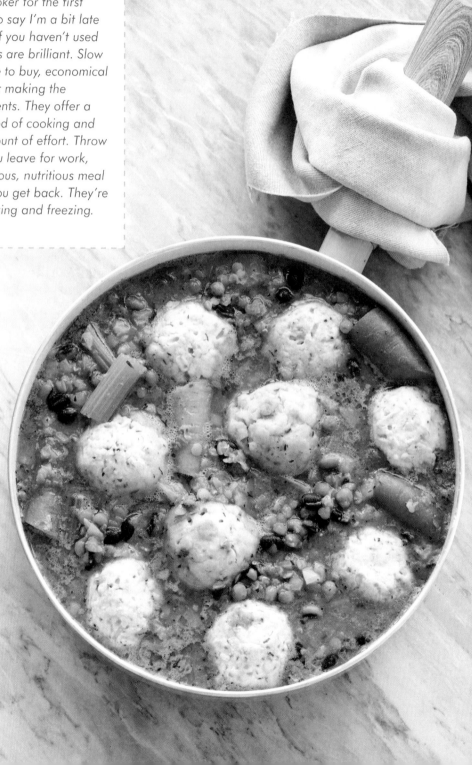

SWEDE STEW
& herby dumplings

This stew is undoubtedly my autumn/winter obsession. As soon as the cooler weather hits, I'm bulk making it like it's going out of fashion! It's inexpensive, extra healthy and perfect for cooking up in giant batches, then freezing for the week ahead.

Serves 4–6

4 white onions, chopped
2 tablespoons olive oil
Bunch of celery, chopped
3 carrots, peeled and chopped
2 parsnips, peeled and chopped
2 sweet potatoes, peeled and chopped
1 swede, peeled and chopped
400g (14oz) can black beans
400g (14oz) can black-eyed beans
200g (7oz) red lentils
4 tablespoons vegan bouillon
2 tablespoons herbes de Provence
150g (5½oz) frozen peas

FOR THE DUMPLINGS
200g (7oz) self-raising flour (I use gluten-free)
150g (5½oz) vegetable suet
2 tablespoons nutritional yeast
1 tablespoon herbes de Provence
Pinch or two of salt

Sauté the onions with the olive oil in a pan over a low heat for 5–10 minutes, or until soft. Add to the slow cooker.

Add the remaining veg to the slow cooker with the beans, lentils, bouillon and herbs and 2 litres (3½ pints) of water. The only thing to leave until later is the peas. Cook on high for 2 hours and then on low for a further 4 hours (you may need to adapt depending on your slow cooker settings).

To make the dumplings, add all the ingredients to a mixing bowl. Make a well in the centre and pour in 2 tablespoons of water, stir well and then keep adding a little water at a time until the mixture forms a dough.

Shape the dough into eight dumplings by rolling with your hands. Place in the refrigerator until you're ready to cook them.

When your stew needs just half an hour longer, add the peas and dumplings, replace the lid and cook for 30 minutes. Serve.

MEXICAN
bean chilli

As someone who is particularly sensitive to nightshades, I'd assumed Mexican foods were something I'd have to exclude from my diet for good. That was until I created my tomato-less sauce that, combined with herbs and cacao, provides a warm and earthy Mexican chilli base. Another brilliant bulk prep recipe, perfect for warming up on cold winter evenings.

Serves 4–6

4 white onions, chopped
2 tablespoons olive oil
2 × 400g (14oz) cans kidney beans, drained
2 × 400g (14oz) cans mixed beans, drained
200g (7oz) can sweetcorn, drained
500ml (18fl oz) Tomato-less Sauce (see page 61)
300g (10½oz) chopped mushrooms
1 garlic clove, crushed
2 tablespoons balsamic vinegar
2 tablespoons vegan bouillon
1 teaspoon dried oregano
2 teaspoons cacao powder
1 tablespoon black pepper
1 teaspoon ground cumin
1 teaspoon ground cinnamon

TO SERVE
Juice of ½ lime
Fresh coriander (cilantro), chopped

Sauté the onions with the olive oil in a pan over a low heat for 5–10 minutes, or until soft, then add to the slow cooker.

Add the remaining ingredients to the slow cooker with 1 litre (1¾ pints) of water. Cook on medium for 6 hours (you may need to adapt depending on your slow cooker settings).

Serve with lime juice and fresh coriander (cilantro).

SWEET POTATO
slow-cooker curry

When it comes to bulk prepping family favourites, everybody loves a curry. This healthy recipe is the perfect alternative to a Friday night takeaway and it can be bulk prepped to be on the table in less time than it will take you to dial in your order!

Serves 4–6

1 tablespoon coconut oil
1 onion, diced
2 medium sweet potatoes, peeled and cubed
400g (14oz) can chickpeas, drained
500ml (18fl oz) Tomato-less Sauce (see page 61)
100g (3½oz) red lentils
4 garlic cloves, minced
2 tablespoons curry powder
2 teaspoons ground cumin
1 tablespoon garam masala (blend without chillies)
500ml (18fl oz) water
2 tablespoons vegan bouillon

TO SERVE
Fresh coriander (cilantro), chopped
Juice of ½ a lemon

Warm the coconut oil in a pan over a low heat and sauté the onion for 5–7 minutes until soft. Add the onion and all the remaining ingredients to your slow cooker. Give it a good stir, then cook on low for 6–8 hours.
Serve with freshly chopped coriander (cilantro) and fresh lemon juice.

BUTTERNUT
squash tagine

I find sweet, plump apricots and tender butternut squash to be a winner with toddlers and teens. This delicious Middle Eastern family favourite is fragrantly spiced with the action of slow cooking, giving all the Moroccan flavours lots of time to develop.

Serves 4–6

2 white onions, chopped
2 tablespoons olive oil
1 butternut squash, peeled, deseeded and cubed
500ml (18fl oz) Tomato-less Sauce (see page 61)
3 tablespoons vegan bouillon
4 carrots, peeled and chopped
400g (14oz) can chickpeas
2 garlic cloves, crushed
2 tablespoons maple syrup
10 dried apricots
1 teaspoon ground cinnamon
1 teaspoon ground cumin
1 teaspoon ground coriander
1 teaspoon ground turmeric
½ teaspoon ground ginger
½ teaspoon ground cloves
½ teaspoon ground allspice
Handful of fresh mint, chopped
Handful of fresh parsley, chopped
Handful of fresh coriander (cilantro), chopped, plus extra to serve
Zest and juice of 1 lemon
Salt and black pepper

You can make this recipe in your slow cooker, or if you'd prefer to cook it the traditional way, use an oven tagine.

Sauté the onions with the olive oil in a pan over a low heat for 5–10 minutes, or until soft, then add to the slow cooker.

Add the remaining ingredients, except the fresh herbs and lemon juice, with 1 litre (1¾ pints) of water. Cook on high for 4 hours (you may need to adapt depending on your slow cooker settings).

Finally, stir through the fresh herbs and leave to cook for another 15–30 minutes. Serve with lime juice and fresh coriander (cilantro).

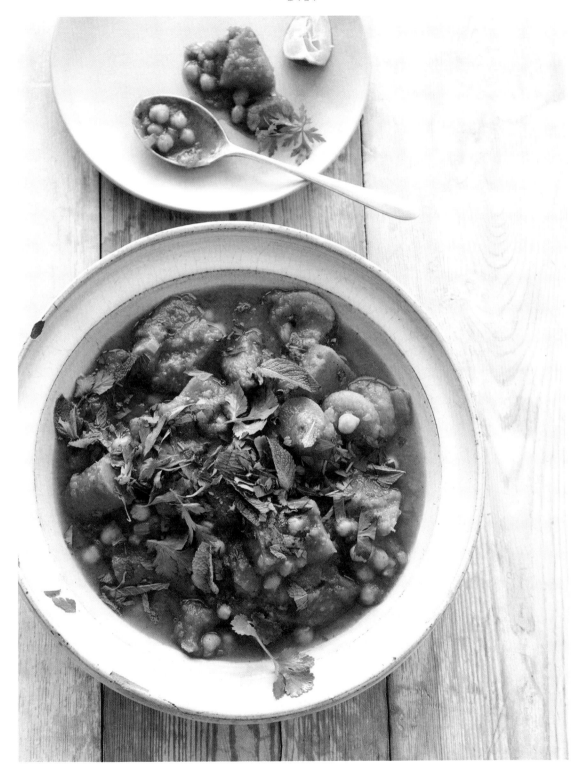

{ pasta and gnocchi }

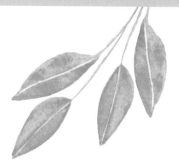

PASTA

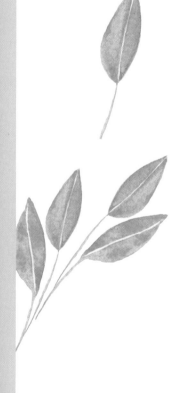

Pasta was always such a quick and simple go-to option. My heart loved it but my belly and brain simply didn't. Wheat pasta would make me feel so bloated and lethargic. I enjoyed eating it but hated the feeling afterwards. When I first excluded wheat, dairy and nightshades from my diet, I assumed my love affair with tomatoey pasta dishes and creamy mac 'n' cheese was done!

Over the past year alone, gluten-free pasta has become so much more widely available in the supermarkets. It has massively dropped in price recently and actually cooks so well and tastes so good that you'd have trouble distinguishing it from the wheat version. Rice pasta, maize pasta, lentil pasta, chickpea pasta, edamame bean pasta, even seaweed pasta! The alternatives on offer are endless.

If your local supermarket does not stock an alternative, or if you'd like to add even more plant-powered goodness to your meal, a spiralizer or mandolin quickly turns ordinary sweet potatoes, courgettes (zucchini) and parsnips into "pasta" ribbons. I also love to make gluten- and potato-free gnocchi using root vegetables and rice flour.

Whether I go for packet pasta or freshly prepared vegetable ribbons usually depends on how much time I have. Frozen sauces and packet pasta can keep you on track when you're home late from work and need a quick ready-made go-to.

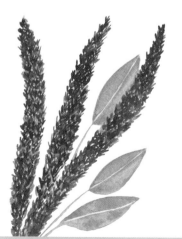

TOMATO-LESS *sauce*

Out of all the things I changed in my diet, I never realized how much I'd miss tomatoes!

My tomato-less sauce is a game changer when it comes to excluding nightshades. Having a simple substitute for canned tomatoes means I can cook from lots of mainstream vegan recipe books again. Variety is key when it comes to keeping a new regime interesting. Best of all, this recipe requires little effort to make and freezes really well. I freeze batches in silicone muffin trays and simply pop out a portion when a recipe calls for tomatoes.

Makes approximately 1.5 litres (2½ pints)

  2 onions, chopped
  2 leeks, chopped
  4 carrots, peeled and chopped
  1 beetroot, peeled and chopped
  5 celery sticks, chopped
  2 garlic cloves, chopped
  3 tablespoons vegan bouillon
  3 lemons

Add the vegetables to a saucepan. Fill a jug with 1.5 litres (2½ pints) boiled water and stir in the vegan bouillon. Pour the water over the chopped vegetables until it rises just above them. Simmer for 1 hour over a gentle heat, or until the beets have softened.

Allow to cool, then ladle the vegetables into a high-speed blender and blitz as you would soup.

Once everything in the pan is blended smooth, begin to add lemon juice to taste, to create an acidic tang.

Store in the refrigerator for 2–3 days or in the freezer for up to 3 months.

NOTE

If you find your sauce is too pink, add more carrots and reduce the quantity of beets in future. If you can't find raw beetroot, precooked will give you the same reddish pink colour but doesn't taste quite as earthy.

VARIATIONS

Once you've mastered this base recipe, you can experiment with a whole variety of sauces that are usually tomato-based by adding the ingredients below to taste:

- Add coconut sugar and salt, a teaspoon at a time, to create a thick tomato ketchup.
- Add hickory smoke, cumin powder, tamari sauce and balsamic vinegar to create a smoky BBQ sauce.
- Add extra crushed garlic, black pepper, dried oregano and basil to make a fresh Italian sauce.
- Add ground coriander, cumin, turmeric, ginger, fennel seeds, ground cardamom, star anise and black pepper to create a warming curry sauce.

GARDEN PEA, COURGETTE
& mint pesto pasta

If you're up for starting a little herb garden at home, you can't go wrong with mint! This stuff spreads like wildfire, smells delicious and is great for adding to juices, teas and sauces. I had so much fresh mint growing in my garden over the summer, I was searching for new recipes to use it all up. That's where I stumbled upon the idea of mint pesto. This dish is a zingy pasta favourite with a fresh take on a traditional basil pesto.

Serves 2

150g (5¼oz) pasta (I use gluten-free spaghetti)
1 large courgette (zucchini)
1 tablespoon olive oil
100g (3½oz) garden peas
A small handful of mint leaves, finely sliced
100g (3½oz) vegan feta, crumbled (optional)
Squeeze of lemon juice
Salt and black pepper
Fresh parsley, chopped, to garnish

FOR THE PESTO
3 large handfuls of fresh mint
Handful of fresh parsley
Juice of 1 lemon
100ml (3½fl oz) extra virgin olive oil
1 garlic clove, peeled
75g (2¾oz) blanched almonds
2 tablespoons nutritional yeast

Cook the pasta in a pan of boiling salted water according to the packet instructions, then drain.

Meanwhile, slice the courgettes (zucchini) lengthways with a sharp knife or using a mandolin.

Place a frying pan over a medium heat with 1 tablespoon of olive oil, then add the courgettes (zucchini) and peas. Cook for 4 minutes, tossing regularly.

Meanwhile, add all the pesto ingredients to a food-processor or mini chopper and pulse, scraping down the sides to combine everything together well.

Stir the mint leaves into the greens. Toss the pasta into the courgette (zucchini) pan and season with salt and pepper. Finally, spoon in the mint pesto and continue to stir everything through.

Dish up with crumbled feta (if using), a squeeze of fresh lemon and some finely chopped parsley.

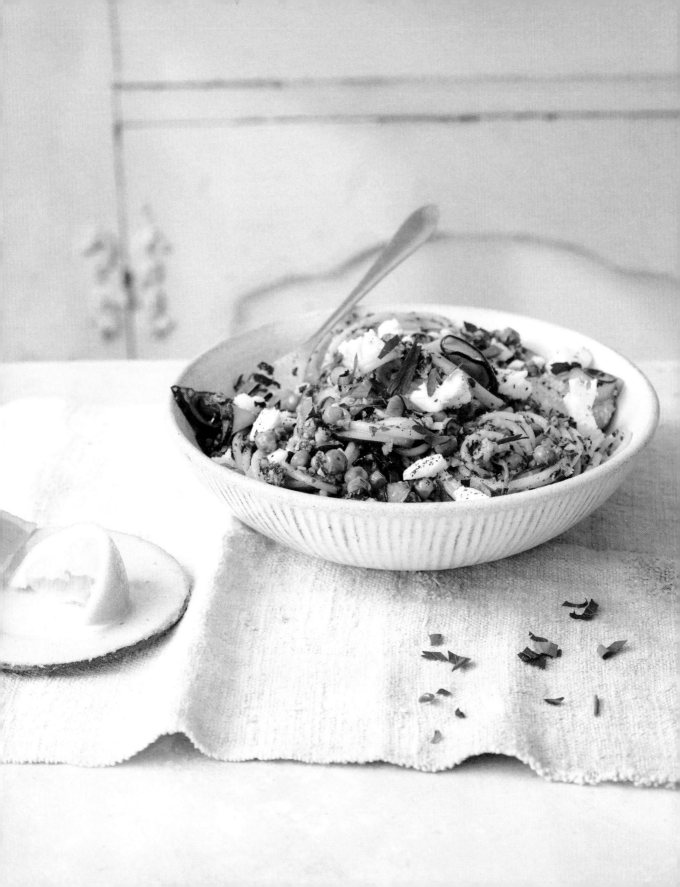

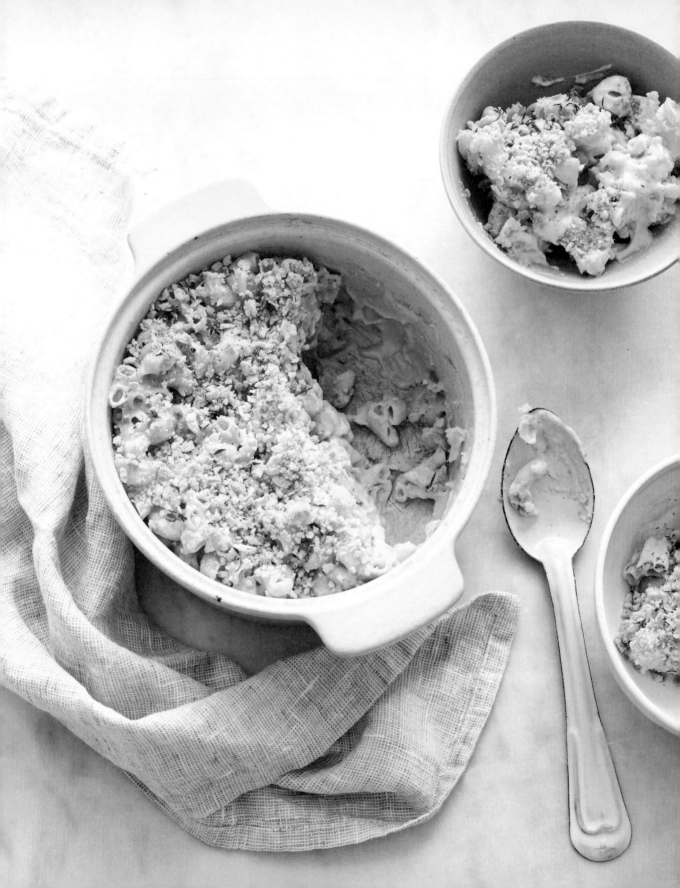

VEGAN *mac 'n' cheese*

With so many dairy-free cheese alternatives gradually making their way on to our supermarket shelves, mac and cheese is firmly back on the menu for us vegans. Wonderfully rich and comforting, this recipe makes a brilliant quick lunch or dinner option.

Serves 2

150g (5½oz) cashews
200ml (7fl oz) boiling water
150g (5½oz) macaroni (I use gluten-free)
3 tablespoons nutritional yeast
Juice of 1 lemon
1 tablespoon apple cider vinegar
1 teaspoon English mustard
2 fresh thyme sprigs
20g (¾oz) breadcrumbs (I use gluten-free)
Salt and black pepper

Soak the cashews by adding them to a blending cup and covering with the boiling water for 30 minutes.

Preheat the oven to 180°C/350°F/gas mark 4.

Meanwhile, cook the macaroni in a pan of boiling salted water according to the packet instructions, then drain.

Spoon 2 tablespoons of the nutritional yeast, lemon juice, mustard, apple cider vinegar and a pinch of salt to the soaked cashews and blitz until smooth. Add the macaroni to this cashew sauce and toss to coat, before spooning it into an ovenproof dish.

Pick the thyme leaves and add them to a bowl with the remaining nutritional yeast and the breadcrumbs. Combine well and sprinkle over the pasta. Place the dish in a hot oven for around 20 minutes, or until golden and bubbling.

Leave to stand for 5 minutes, then serve with seasonal greens.

PARSNIP *gnocchi*

This is such a super-easy alternative to potato gnocchi. It lends itself brilliantly to a variety of pasta sauces and toppings. As a shortcut you can skip the bit where you fry the gnocchi off after boiling it, but this way of cooking it was recommended to me by a chef many years ago, and it's so good, I've prepared it like this ever since.

Serves 2

400g (14oz) parsnips, peeled and cut into chunks
4 tablespoons olive oil
1 garlic clove
100g (3½oz) plain flour (I use gluten-free)
½ teaspoon grated nutmeg
4 heaped tablespoons nutritional yeast
Salt and black pepper
Truffle oil, to serve

KALE PESTO
30g (1oz) pine nuts, toasted
30g (1oz) walnuts, toasted and chopped
2 tablespoons nutritional yeast
2 garlic cloves, peeled
60ml (2fl oz) olive oil
85g (3oz) kale
Juice of 1 lemon

Preheat the oven to 180°C/350°F/gas mark 4.

Toss the parsnips in 2 tablespoons of the olive oil and tip into a roasting tin along with the garlic clove. Roast for 40 minutes, or until soft.

Add to a food processor along with the flour, nutmeg and nutritional yeast, season well, then pulse until combined and holding together as a dough. Roll the dough into long sausages between your hands. Place on a floured surface and cut each sausage into small, pillow-shaped gnocchi, each around 2cm (¾ inch) long.

Boil a pan of salted water and add the gnocchi in batches for 1 minute, or until they float to the surface. Remove from the water with a slotted spoon and drain.

Heat the remaining olive oil in a frying pan over a medium heat. Add the gnocchi and fry until lightly golden on each side, around 3–4 minutes. You might need to do this in batches depending on the size of your pan.

To make the pesto, put the pine nuts, walnuts, nutritional yeast, garlic, oil, kale and lemon juice in a food processor and whizz to a paste. Season to taste.

When all the gnocchi are golden, return them all to the pan to warm through before dividing between two plates. Sprinkle over some black pepper and serve with kale walnut pesto and a drizzle of truffle oil.

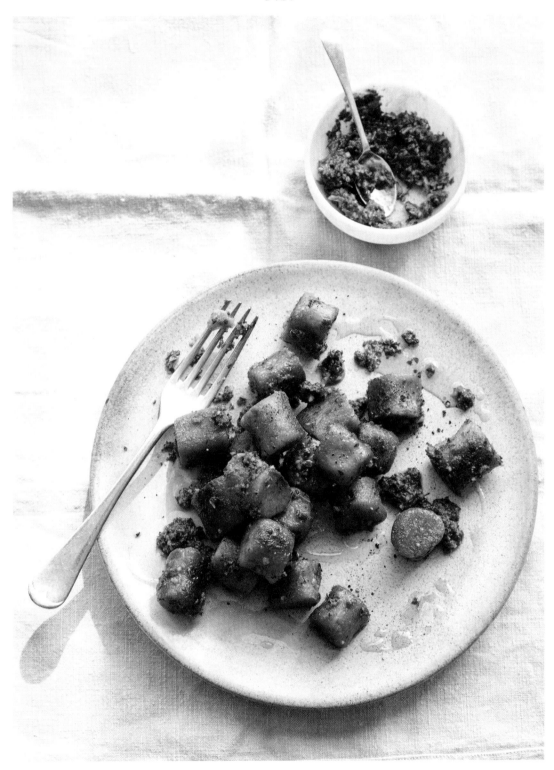

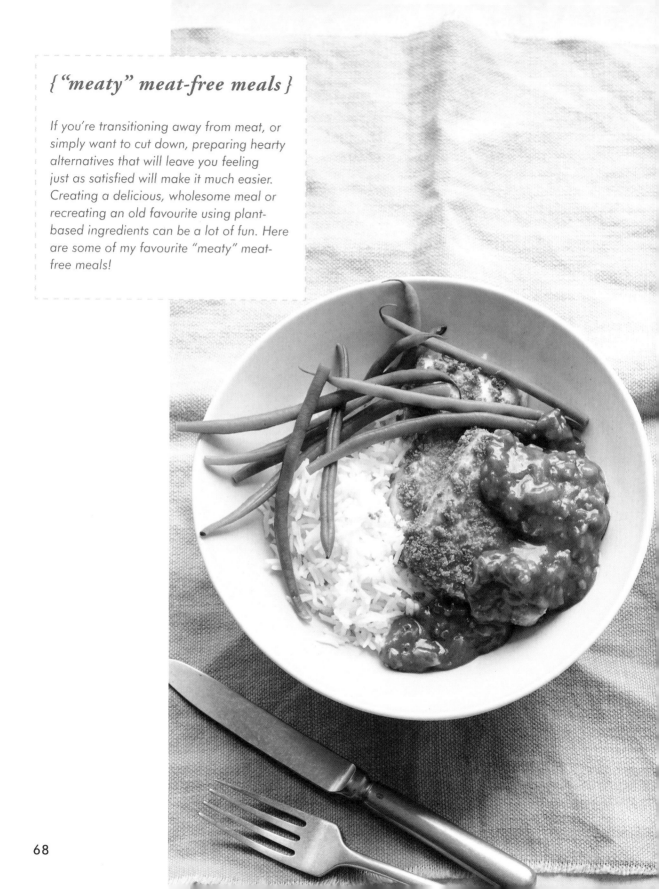

{ "meaty" meat-free meals }

If you're transitioning away from meat, or simply want to cut down, preparing hearty alternatives that will leave you feeling just as satisfied will make it much easier. Creating a delicious, wholesome meal or recreating an old favourite using plant-based ingredients can be a lot of fun. Here are some of my favourite "meaty" meat-free meals!

BREADED TOFU
katsu curry

This is my vegan version of the delicious Japanese katsu curry they serve at Wagamama. I was so ridiculously excited when I found out I didn't need tomatoes to make this dish and I honestly could not believe how simple it is to get the flavour absolutely spot on.

Serves 2

2 tablespoons coconut oil
2 white onions, finely chopped
1 carrot, finely chopped
2.5cm (1 inch) piece of fresh root ginger, peeled and grated
1 garlic clove, crushed
1 tablespoon garam masala
2 heaped tablespoons flour (I use gluten-free)
2 tablespoons vegan bouillon dissolved in 500ml (17fl oz) water
1 tablespoon tamari
1 tablespoon maple syrup
400g (14oz) tofu
3 tablespoons vegan mayonnaise
50g (1¾oz) gluten-free breadcrumbs
Cooked rice and green beans, to serve

Sauté the onions in 1 tablespoon of the coconut oil over a low heat for a couple of minutes. Add the carrot, ginger and garlic and sweat over a low heat for 10 minutes. I pop a lid on the pan and let everything slowly soften.

Add the garam masala and flour and stir well. Now it's time to gradually pour in the warm stock. Do it slowly, a bit at a time, and keep stirring well as you do so.

Flavour with tamari and maple syrup. You'll want to do this to your taste, so gradually keep adding a little of each until you're happy with the flavour. Now you can either strain the sauce to remove the carrots and onions, or leave them in if you prefer.

While the sauce is warming, split the tofu into two evenly sized "steaks". Brush each one with vegan mayonnaise and coat in breadcrumbs. Heat the remaining coconut oil in a pan over a medium heat and fry the breaded tofu steaks for around 5 minutes on each side until crisp and golden.

To serve, pour the sauce over the breaded tofu steaks and serve with rice and green beans.

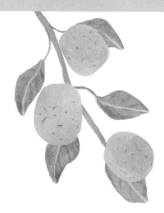

JACKFRUIT

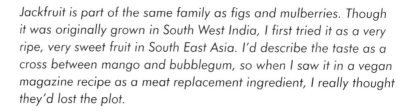

Jackfruit is part of the same family as figs and mulberries. Though it was originally grown in South West India, I first tried it as a very ripe, very sweet fruit in South East Asia. I'd describe the taste as a cross between mango and bubblegum, so when I saw it in a vegan magazine recipe as a meat replacement ingredient, I really thought they'd lost the plot.

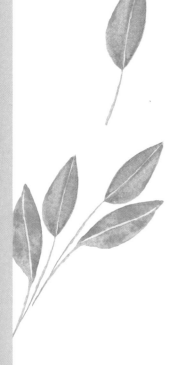

The outside of the jackfruit is all green and spiky; inside the fruit is yellow in colour – similar to, but a little bit paler than, mango. Unripened jackfruit has a sort of stringy consistency, and it's nowhere near as sweet as the ripe version, which is why you'll often find unripened jackfruit suggested in recipes and used in ready-meals as a plant-based version of shredded chicken, pulled pork or other meats.

Once a mystical ingredient that you could only find online or in Asian and Indian food shops, canned jackfruit is now much more readily available on supermarket shelves. You can even buy prepared shredded versions at some of the larger stores.

My favourite way to cook jackfruit is by warming a little oil in a pan and heating the chunks until they begin to soften and can easily be pulled apart with a fork to create a shredded texture. Unripened jackfruit is pretty flavourless, which is great, because it means you can use sauces and spices to flavour it as you wish.

Here are two of my favourite jackfruit recipes. Pulled jackfruit is now a firm fixture on vegan menus, and this clever "pulled" meat substitute is easy to make at home, perfect for stuffing into bread rolls and enjoying with all the barbecue trimmings. My jackfruit "tuna" melt is another great option, and is virtually indistinguishable from the real thing. The way it looks, the taste and the texture are quite amazing – one of my absolute favourite sandwiches ever!

JACKFRUIT
"tuna" melt

Serves 2

1 tablespoon olive oil
565g (20oz) can young, green jackfruit
 in brine, drained and rinsed
1 teaspoon kelp powder (or crushed
 seaweed sheet)
200g (7oz) can sweetcorn, drained
3 tablespoons vegan mayo
4 slices sourdough bread
2 slices vegan cheese
Salt and black pepper

Preheat the grill to medium/high.

Heat the oil in a large pan, add the drained jackfruit and cook over a medium–low heat for 10 minutes. As it begins to soften, use a fork to shred the jackfruit apart.

Add the kelp powder or crushed seaweed sheet and stir through. Turn off the heat and stir the sweetcorn and mayonnaise through the jackfruit, then season with salt and pepper.

Toast the sourdough slices under the grill for 2 minutes.

Spoon the jackfruit mayo on to two of the sourdough slices, add a slice of vegan cheese on top and grill for another minute or two until melted. Add the second toasted slice on top, slice in half and serve.

PULLED
jackfruit in a bun

Serves 2

1 tablespoon olive oil
1 red onion, finely chopped
565g (20oz) can young, green jackfruit
 in brine, drained and rinsed
100ml (3½fl oz) Tomato-less BBQ Sauce
 (see Variations on page 61), plus extra
 to serve
2 burger buns (I use gluten-free)
Salt and black pepper

Heat the oil in a large pan. When it's hot, add the chopped onion and cook over a low–medium heat for 5–7 minutes, or until the onion softens. Add the drained jackfruit and cook over a medium–low heat for 10 minutes. As it begins to soften, use a fork to shred the jackfruit apart.

Add the Tomato-less BBQ sauce and continue to stir over a low heat for a further 10 minutes, until sticky and well combined. Season and spoon on to burger buns. Serve with extra sauce.

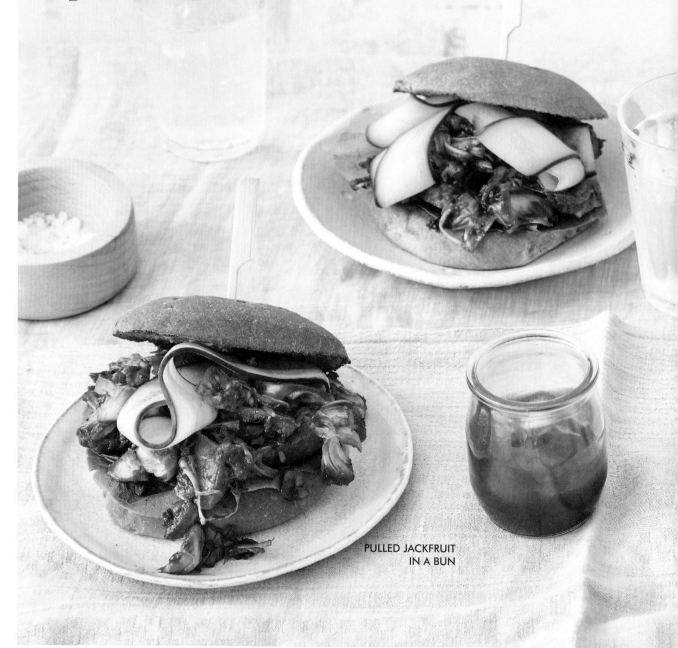

Unripened jackfruit can be used as a plant-based substitute for shredded chicken, pulled pork or other meats

PULLED JACKFRUIT
IN A BUN

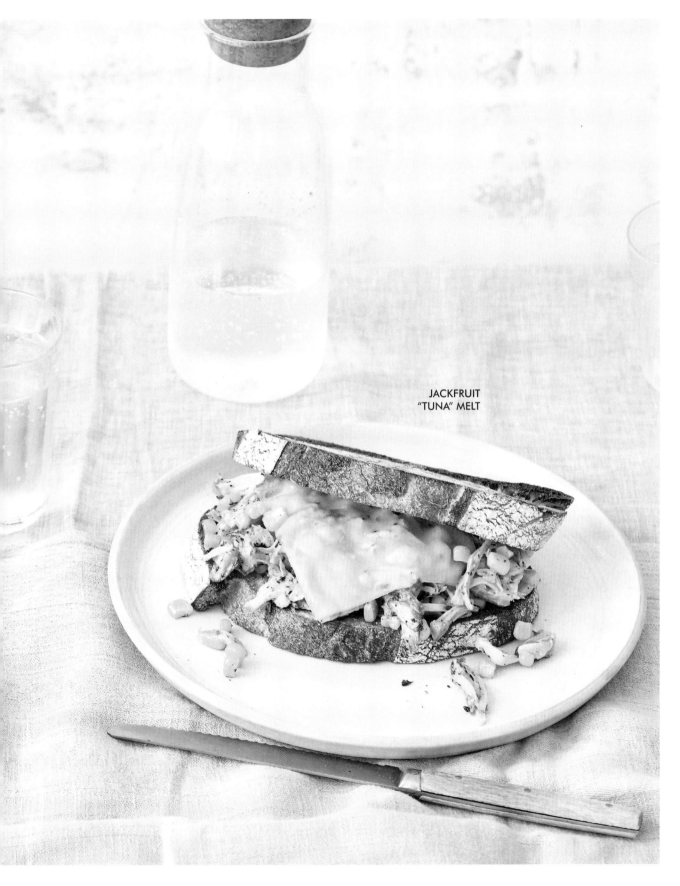

JACKFRUIT
"TUNA" MELT

TEMPEH VEGAN
BBQ "ribs"

This plant-based version of a classic American favourite will surely be the hit of your next barbecue. Meaty, smoky and super sticky, it has all the textures and flavours we love. While most of these ingredients are easy to find in the supermarket, liquid hickory smoke is one you'll need to order online. It's absolutely worth it if you love that authentic smoky flavour in your cooking.

Serves 2

3 tablespoons tamari sauce
1 tablespoon maple syrup
1 teaspoon liquid hickory smoke
½ teaspoon onion powder
½ teaspoon garlic powder
2 tablespoons coconut oil
200g (7oz) block of tempeh
250ml (9fl oz) Tomato-less BBQ Sauce (see Variations on page 61)

Preheat the oven to 180°C/350°F/gas mark 4.

Whisk 60ml (2fl oz) water together with the tamari sauce, maple syrup, liquid hickory smoke, onion powder and garlic powder in a bowl.

Melt the coconut oil in a medium frying pan over a medium heat. Carefully place the entire block of tempeh into the pan and pour over the tamari sauce mixture. Bring the liquid to a simmer. Allow the liquid to simmer for about 5 minutes, flip the tempeh, and then allow it to simmer for another 5 minutes. Remove from the heat and brush on half the BBQ sauce.

Place on a baking tray and bake for about 5–10 minutes.

Slice the tempeh into strips and serve with the remaining BBQ sauce on the side.

CHICKPEA
nuggets

This is such a fab recipe for kids and adults alike. Great for quick dipping snacks or loading up on to your child's plate for extra protein.

Serves 2

400g (14oz) can chickpeas, drained
75g (2¾oz) plain flour (I use gluten-free)
100g (3½oz) gluten-free breadcrumbs
3 tablespoons vegan mayonnaise
Pinch of garlic salt
1 teaspoon mixed Italian herbs
1 tablespoon olive oil
2 tablespoons coconut oil, for frying
Salt
Tomato-less BBQ Sauce (see Variations on
     page 61), to serve

Add everything except the coconut oil to the food processor and pulse together. You might need to stir with a spoon part way through to ensure the mixture is evenly combined.

Form into little nugget shapes. Brush each one in mayonnaise and then dip into the breadcrumbs before popping in the refrigerator for 30 minutes.

Heat the coconut oil in a pan over a low–medium heat and fry the nuggets for 5 minutes on each side until crisp and golden. Serve with BBQ sauce.

A fab recipe for kids and adults alike

SEASONED
cauli steaks

Make no mistake, meatless "steaks" don't mean they're not hearty, filling or super delicious. Inexpensive, easy to make, healthy and extra satisfying, they're perfect served with steamed veg or a fresh summer salad.

Serves 2

1 cauliflower, middle section
   sliced into two 2.5-cm (1-inch) steaks
2 tablespoons olive oil
1 teaspoon ground cumin
1 teaspoon ground coriander
6 shallots, finely sliced
30g (1oz) pine nuts, toasted
2 garlic cloves, finely chopped
1 teaspoon cumin seeds
Zest and juice of ½ lemon
Handful of fresh parsley, chopped
Salt
Steamed green beans, to serve

Preheat the oven to 200°C/400°F/gas mark 6 and line a baking tray with greaseproof paper.

Rub 1 tablespoon of oil, plus the cumin and coriander, over the cauliflower steaks and season with salt. Place on the tray and roast for 15–20 minutes, or until cooked through.

Meanwhile, put the remaining oil and the shallots into a pan and fry over a medium heat for 2–3 minutes. Add the pine nuts and fry for 3–4 minutes, then add the garlic and cumin seeds and fry for another minute. Add the lemon zest and juice, then season.

Top the cauliflower with the shallots, pine nuts and chopped parsley, and serve immediately with steamed green beans.

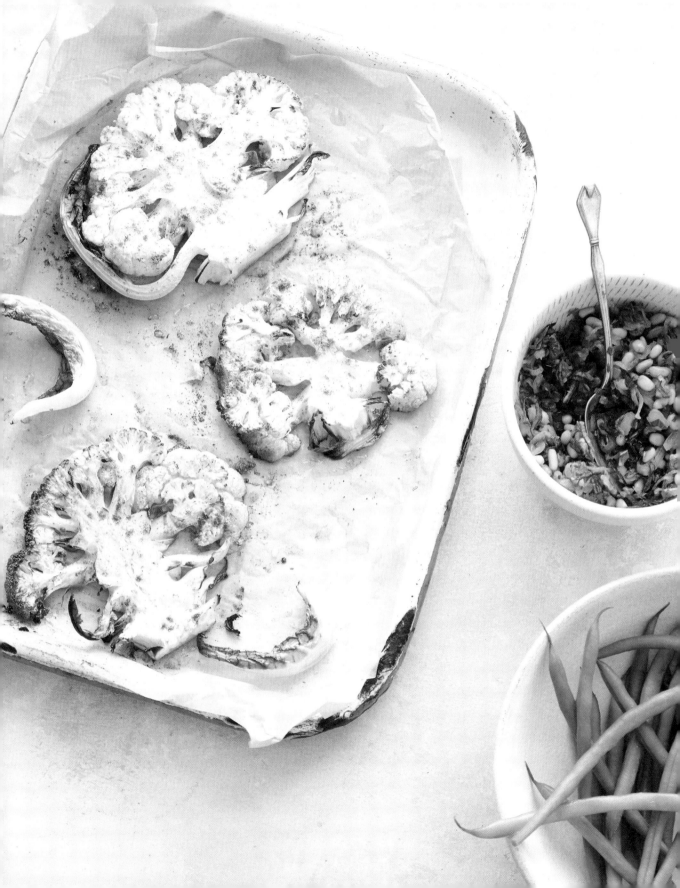

SIMPLE CELERY *soup*

This simple soup recipe is perfect and packed full of flavour. Celery is super-rich in vitamin K, which helps boost blood flow and circulation. It also has a very cooling and refreshing effect, which is great for the skin, particularly if you're wanting to make soup during the hotter months of the year.

Serves 2

1 tablespoon olive oil
1 onion, chopped
1 leek, chopped
2 garlic cloves, crushed
Bunch of celery, chopped
500ml (18fl oz) water
2 tablespoons vegan bouillon
2 bay leaves
Handful of fresh parsley, chopped

Heat the oil in a saucepan over a low heat and sauté the onion for 5 minutes.

Add the leek, garlic and celery and cook over a low heat for a further 5 minutes, or until softened.

Add the water, bouillon and bay leaves, and simmer for 10–12 minutes.

Transfer the soup to a blender and liquidize. Serve with fresh parsley.

> *Celery is super-rich in vitamin K, which helps boost blood flow and circulation*

EARTHY
mushroom soup

Mushroom soup always reminds me of my grandad. He used to prepare steamy, creamy bowls of the stuff for lunch. Rich and filling, this smooth mushroom recipe has intensely earthy flavours. You'll never go back to canned once you've tried this delicious homemade version.

Serves 4

500g (1lb 2oz) mushrooms
4 garlic cloves, chopped
1 medium onion, chopped
750ml (25fl oz) almond milk
2 tablespoons vegan bouillon, dissolved in 500ml (18fl oz) boiling water
1 teaspoon dried tarragon
Pinch of black pepper
Juice of 1 lemon

TO SERVE
Sautéed mushrooms
Fresh parsley, chopped

Set a handful of mushrooms aside and add the rest to a large pot, along with the garlic, onion, almond milk and vegetable stock. Bring to the boil, then simmer over a medium heat for 10 minutes.

Meanwhile, sauté the reserved mushrooms in a little oil and set aside.

Blend the soup with a handheld blender or in a regular blender. Add the tarragon, black pepper and lemon juice, stir and ladle into bowls.

Top with the sautéed mushrooms and chopped fresh parsley.

MISO *soup*

This tofu miso soup recipe really packs a punch, with garlic, ginger and spring onions all making a super-flavoursome broth that will definitely warm you up! Miso is rich in essential minerals and a good source of various B vitamins, as well as vitamins E and K, and folic acid. As a fermented food, miso provides the gut with beneficial bacteria that help us to stay healthy, vibrant and happy.

Serves 2

750ml (25fl oz) water
4 tablespoons vegan bouillon
3cm (1¼ inch) piece of fresh root ginger, peeled and finely sliced
2 garlic cloves, finely sliced
2 spring onions (scallions), finely sliced
½ savoy cabbage, shredded
1 carrot, peeled and finely sliced
2 tablespoons miso paste
Tamari sauce
100g (3½oz) silken tofu, cubed

Pour the water into a pan, add the bouillon and bring to the boil. Add the ginger, garlic and spring onions (scallions) to the stock, cover and simmer for 5 minutes.

Add the cabbage and carrot to the pan, cover and simmer for a further 3–4 minutes, or until the cabbage has wilted.

Stir in the miso paste and a good splash of tamari sauce, to taste. Add the tofu and let it stand for a few minutes before serving.

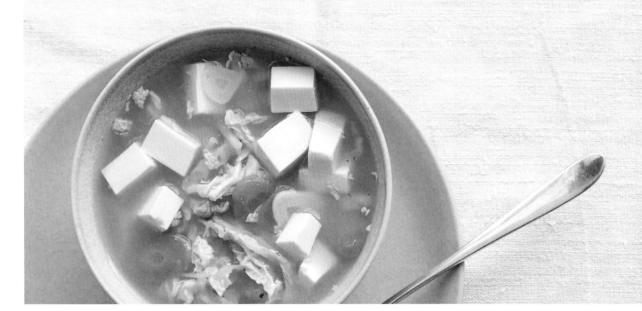

GOLDEN TURMERIC *soup*

*There is so much to be said about the incredible impact turmeric
can have on our skin – see page 108 for why I am such a super fan!
This soup is creamy, wonderfully filling and comes with just the right
amount of spice to offer a warming, hearty lunch.*

Serves 4

1 cauliflower, roughly chopped
2 onions, roughly chopped
1 yellow courgette (zucchini), roughly
   chopped
3 tablespoons olive oil
1 tablespoon ground turmeric
1 tablespoon ground cumin
3 tablespoons vegan bouillon
400g (14oz) can cannellini beans,
   drained
Salt and black pepper

TO GARNISH
Coconut flakes
Ground mixed spice

Preheat the oven to 180°C/350°F/gas mark 4.

Put the cauliflower, onions and courgette (zucchini) in a baking tray. Drizzle in olive oil, then sprinkle with salt and the spices. Oven roast for 30–40 minutes.

Fill a pan with 1.5 litres (2½ pints) of water and bring to the boil, then add the bouillon.

Once the veg is roasted, add it to the pan of stock. Add the can of beans (leave a few to decorate). Turn off the heat and leave to cool.

Pour the soup into a blender and blitz until smooth or use a handheld blender to create a smooth soup.

Garnish with the reserved beans, coconut flakes, black pepper and ground mixed spice.

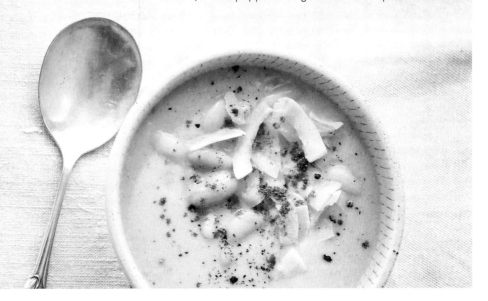

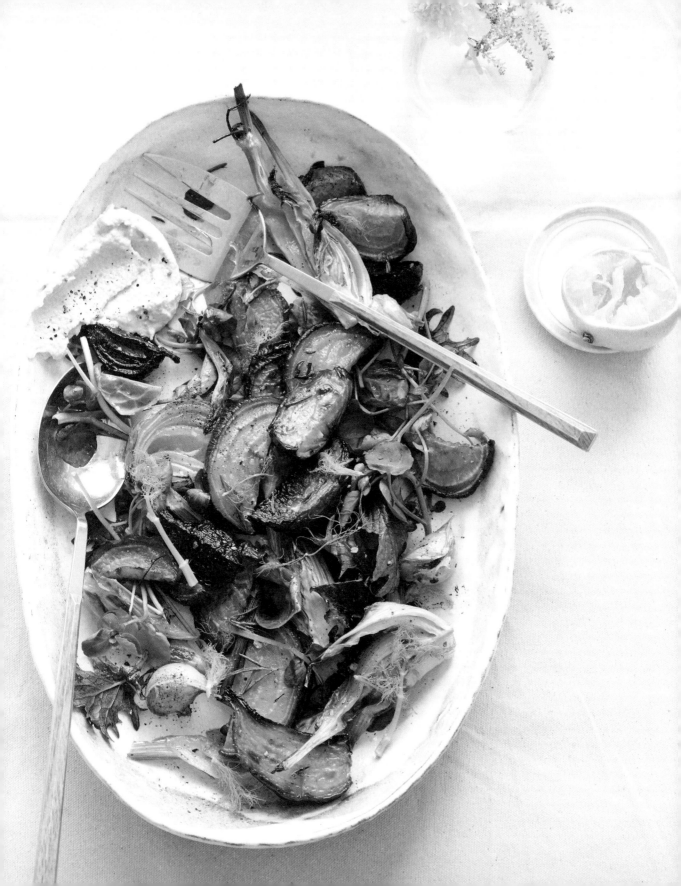

{ salads }

BEETROOT *& fennel salad*

In terms of skin health, beetroot acts as a great blood purifier, which is key in keeping skin glowing and healthy. Beetroot is rich in vitamin C, which helps clear blemishes and evens out skin tone while giving us a natural glow. There are three types of beetroot:

Red beetroots are what most of us think of when our minds turn to beetroot. Look for beetroots with their fresh, leafy greens still attached.

Golden beetroots are a bit less sweet than red beetroots, but also have a more mellow and less earthy flavour all around. If nothing else, golden beetroots add a bright, zesty yellow colour when served roasted or in salads.

Chioggia beetroots are naturally striped. Some are a subtle yellow-and-orange combination while others come with a brilliant red-and-cream candy cane effect.

Serves 2

3 large beetroots, washed well and chopped into large chunks
1 small white onion, quartered
1 bulb fennel, chopped into chunks and fronds reserved
4 garlic cloves
2 tablespoons olive oil
½ teaspoon dried rosemary
½ teaspoon dried thyme
Salt and black pepper

TO SERVE
Salad leaves
Hummus
Juice of ½ lemon

Preheat the oven to 180°C/350°F/gas mark 4.

Add the beets to a roasting tin with the onion and fennel bulb. Add whole cloves of garlic to the tray. Drizzle in olive oil and sprinkle over rosemary, thyme and salt. Oven roast for about 1 hour (I don't like my beets too soft, but you might want to roast for longer).

Add to a bowl with fresh salad leaves. Spoon on some fresh hummus. Drizzle in fresh lemon juice and grind pepper over the dish. Sprinkle the reserved fennel fronds over to garnish.

SUPER GREEN
detox salad

If you're in need of an extra healthy detox boost, this is the perfect recipe. Filled with heaps of skin-nourishing greens and healthy beneficial oils, then drizzled in the perfect green goodness dressing, it makes for an ideal cleanse option.

Serves 2

140g (5oz) kale, chopped
Olive oil, for massaging
Handful of sugar snap peas
4 broccoli florets
60g (2oz) cooked edamame beans
1 avocado
2 tablespoons sunflower seeds
2 tablespoons pumpkin seeds

FOR THE DRESSING
1 tablespoon olive oil
1 tablespoon tamari
½ tablespoon maple syrup
Large handful of fresh coriander (cilantro), chopped
Large handful of fresh parsley, chopped
½ teaspoon salt
½ teaspoon black pepper

Massage the chopped kale with a little olive oil and a pinch of salt. Rub with your fingers until the leaves begin to darken and tenderize. This makes it taste great and gives the kale a silky texture.

Add to a salad bowl along with the peas, broccoli and edamame beans.

Combine all the dressing ingredients in a small bowl. Stir through the salad and top with fresh avocado and seeds to serve.

*If you're in need
of an extra healthy
detox boost, this is the
perfect recipe*

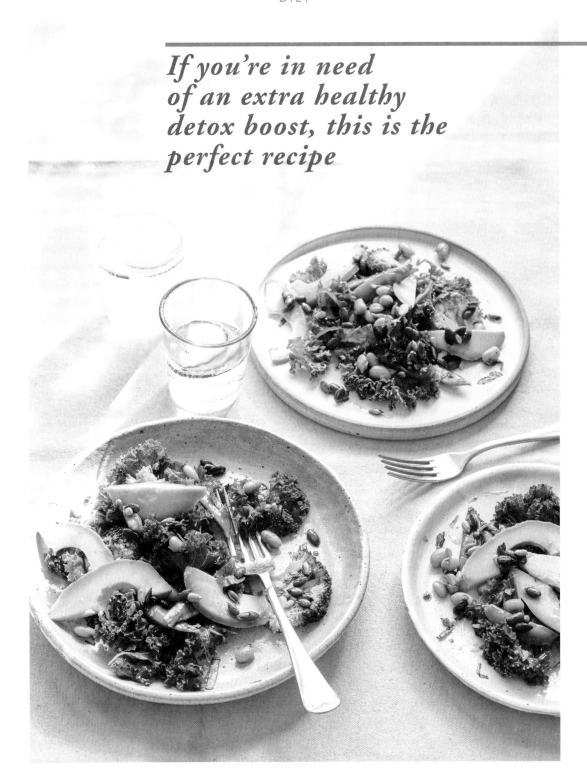

APPLE *& walnut salad*

The perfect mix of sweet, zesty and crunchy.

Serves 2

½ romaine lettuce, leaves separated
½ red leaf lettuce, chopped
1 red and 1 green apple, chopped
100g (3½oz) walnuts, chopped
50g (1¾oz) dried cranberries

FOR THE VINAIGRETTE
75ml (2½fl oz) extra virgin olive oil
1 tablespoon balsamic vinegar
2 teaspoons maple syrup
1 tablespoon wholegrain mustard
Salt and black pepper

In a large bowl combine the lettuce, apples, walnuts and cranberries. Combine all the ingredients for the vinaigrette, then drizzle over the salad and toss to combine. Serve.

ROAST CARROT, RADISH *& raisin salad*

A hearty salad with so much colour and flavour it makes a meal in itself.

Serves 2

6 small carrots, peeled and chopped
8 radishes, halved
400g (14oz) can chickpeas, drained
1 red onion, finely chopped
Juice of ½ lemon
2 teaspoons ground cinnamon
1 teaspoon ground cumin
1 tablespoon extra virgin olive oil
1 garlic clove, grated
100g (3½oz) rocket (arugula)
50g (1¾oz) pitted dates, finely diced
1 tablespoon toasted flaked almonds
Salt
Coconut yogurt, to serve

Preheat the oven to 180°C/350°F/gas mark 4 and line a baking tray with greaseproof paper.

Place the carrots in a bowl along with the radishes, drained chickpeas, red onion, lemon juice, spices, olive oil, salt and garlic. Toss well to coat evenly. Spread out in a single layer on the baking tray and roast for 25–30 minutes, or until tender and slightly caramelized. Set aside to cool.

Place the rocket (arugula) in a serving bowl or platter. Top with the carrot and chickpea mixture. Sprinkle with dates and the toasted flaked almonds and serve with coconut yogurt.

COURGETTE, QUINOA
& fresh mint salad

I've had an endless supply of home-grown courgettes (zucchini) this year! I started out a little disappointed as the garden snails were getting to them before I was. But gradually, as the plants grew tougher, they yielded an awesome crop. The flowers, young leaves and even the shoot tips of the courgette plant are all edible, and the courgettes themselves make for delicious summer salads such as this one.

Serves 2

1 tablespoon vegan boullion
200g (7oz) quinoa
2 large courgettes (zucchini)
1 tablespoon olive oil
50g (1¾oz) pitted black olives
Juice of ½ lemon
1 tablespoon maple syrup
2 teaspoons cumin seeds
1 garlic clove, crushed (use fermented garlic for a softer taste, see page 101)
Salt and black pepper

FOR THE COCONUT YOGURT DRESSING
100g (3½oz) coconut yogurt
Handful of fresh mint, chopped
Handful of fresh parsley, chopped
Pinch of salt
1 teaspoon maple syrup
Juice of ½ lemon

TO SERVE
100g (3½oz) rocket (arugula)
Handful of fresh mint leaves

Boil a pan of water and add the vegan bouillon powder. Add the quinoa and simmer for 10–15 minutes, or until softened. Drain and set aside.

For the coconut yogurt dressing, mix everything together well and place in the refrigerator until ready to serve.

Meanwhile, slice the courgettes (zucchini) into thin discs. Warm the olive oil in a pan over a low–medium heat, add the courgette (zucchini) discs, sprinkle with salt and lightly fry on each side for a couple of minutes.

Add the quinoa to the pan and season with salt and pepper. Add the olives, lemon juice, maple syrup, cumin seeds and crushed garlic.

Serve on a bed of rocket (arugula) salad with fresh mint leaves and the coconut yogurt dressing.

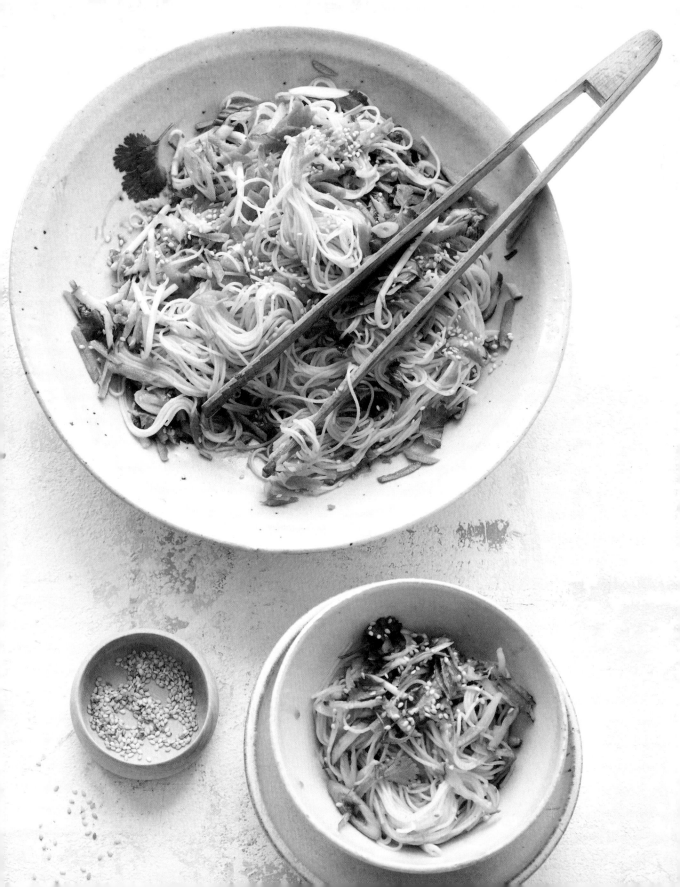

VIETNAMESE
noodle salad

This Asian noodle salad comes with plenty of colourful vegetables and a fresh tamari dressing. A fantastic, vegan, make-ahead lunch that's loaded up with healthy veggies and perfect for individual midweek lunches or bigger shared platters.

Serves 2

200g vermicelli rice noodles
2 carrots, finely grated
2 cucumbers, deseeded and grated
4 spring onions (scallions), finely chopped
100g (3½oz) bean sprouts
Large handful of fresh coriander (cilantro)
100ml (3½fl oz) seasoned rice vinegar
1 tablespoon tamari
3 tablespoons coconut sugar
2 garlic cloves, minced
Juice of 1 lime
2 tablespoons sesame seeds

Place the vermicelli noodles in a large bowl, cover with boiling water and soak for 3–4 minutes, or until tender. Rinse under cold water, drain and transfer to a large bowl.

Add the carrots, cucumbers, spring onions (scallions), bean sprouts and chopped coriander (cilantro) to the noodles.

Shake the rice vinegar, tamari, coconut sugar, garlic and lime juice together in a bottle and pour over the salad. Decorate with sesame seeds.

DIPS

Fresh dips are a fantastic way to add flavour to simple salads. They're also a great lunch box addition, and perfect for simply dipping raw vegetables or corn chips. Dips such as hummus bought prepackaged from the supermarket are not the worst thing on earth if you're pushed for time. The ingredients are generally pretty decent and they taste lovely. But if you're bored of plain old hummus or fancy trying something just a little different, these are some of my favourites for adding colour and flavour to the table.

YELLOW SPLIT PEA HUMMUS
A beautiful bright yellow hummus, with warming, fragrant spices.

Serves 4

200g (7oz) yellow split peas
1 tablespoon vegan bouillon
100ml (3½fl oz) extra virgin olive oil
2 tablespoons tahini
2 garlic cloves, peeled
Juice of 1 lemon, plus extra to serve
1 tablespoon maple syrup
½ teaspoon ground cumin
½ teaspoon ground coriander
¼ teaspoon ground turmeric
½ teaspoon salt

TO SERVE
1 tablespoon chopped fresh parsley
Pinch of cumin seeds
Black pepper

Put the split peas into a pan, cover with water, add the bouillon and bring to the boil. Simmer for 40–45 minutes. Take off the heat and let cool.

Once cool, transfer the split peas to a blender. Add all the other hummus ingredients and blend on high until smooth.

Serve with black pepper, fresh parsley and extra lemon juice.

ROAST BEET BLUSH

With the earthy flavour of roast beets, this beautiful blush dip is super creamy with plenty of flavour. Perfect with tortillas, pittas and veggies, or as a healthy, vibrant sandwich filler.

Serves 4

2 cooked beetroots, peeled and cubed
400g (14oz) can chickpeas, drained
1 small garlic clove, chopped
100ml (3½fl oz) olive oil
2 tablespoons tahini
Juice and zest of ½ lemon
1 tablespoon ground cumin
Sesame seeds and chopped fresh mint, to garnish
Salt and black pepper

Preheat the oven to 200°C/400°F/gas mark 6.

Place the beetroot, chickpeas and garlic on a baking tray. Drizzle over the olive oil and roast for 30–40 minutes, or until the beets have softened.

Add to a food processor along with the remaining ingredients. Blitz everything to combine. Taste and adjust the seasoning as needed, adding more salt, lemon juice or olive oil if needed. If it's too thick, add a bit of water.

Garnish with sesame seeds and chopped mint.

PEA AND MINT DIP

This simple dip is totally tasty and bursting with spring-time freshness. Using frozen peas and fresh mint from the garden means you've always got a healthy dip option on hand.

Serves 4

200g (7oz) frozen peas
Large handful of fresh mint, plus extra leaves to garnish
Zest and juice of ½ lemon
1 garlic clove, peeled
2 tablespoons olive oil, plus extra for drizzling
1 tablespoon coconut yogurt
Salt and black pepper

Bring a pan of water to the boil. Add the peas and boil for 2–3 minutes, then drain and cool.

Pulse the peas in a food processor with the mint, lemon zest and juice, garlic and olive oil.

Season with salt and pepper, stir in a spoonful of coconut yogurt, drizzle with extra oil and add some fresh mint leaves.

dips continue on page 94 »

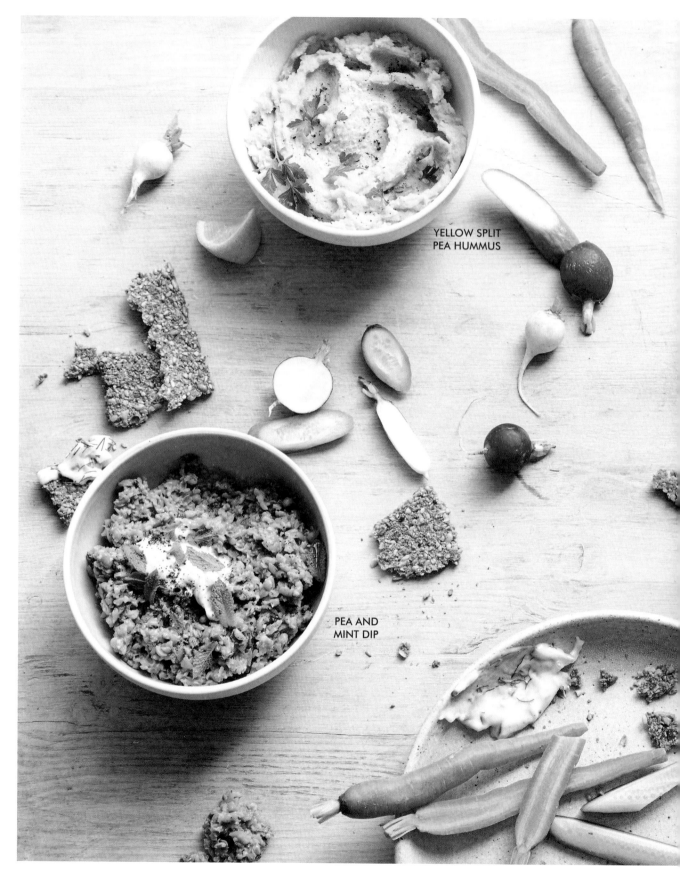

YELLOW SPLIT
PEA HUMMUS

PEA AND
MINT DIP

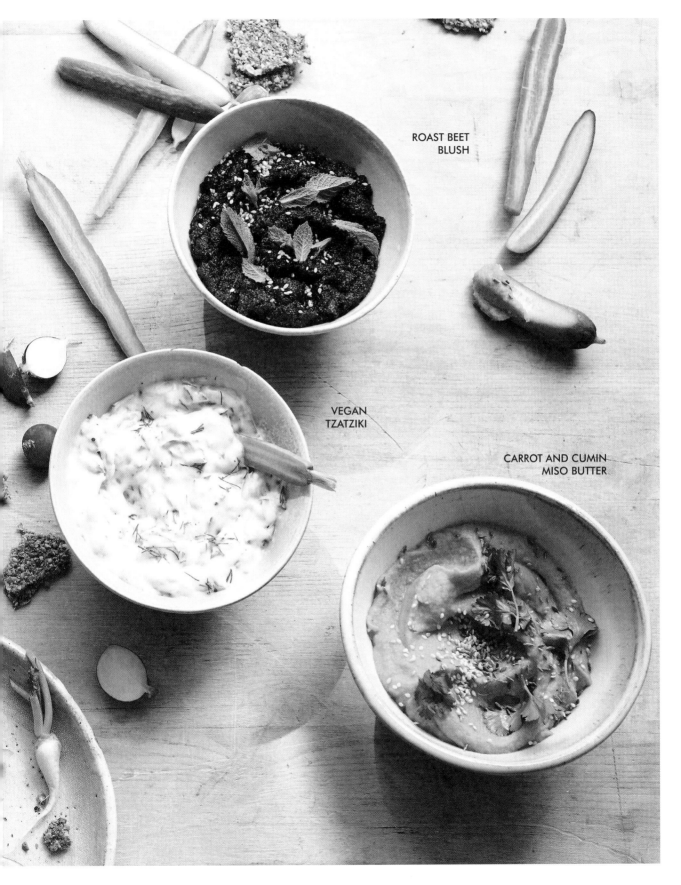

ROAST BEET
BLUSH

VEGAN
TZATZIKI

CARROT AND CUMIN
MISO BUTTER

« dips continued

VEGAN TZATZIKI

This authentic-tasting vegan tzatziki is like no other. Creamy, garlicky and perfect for dipping, this recipe is also delicious on sourdough toast or over falafel.

Serves 4

½ cucumber
200g (7oz) coconut yogurt
3 garlic cloves, minced
Large handful of fresh dill, finely chopped
Pinch of salt
Pinch of black pepper
Juice of ½ lemon
1 teaspoon maple syrup

Finely grate the cucumber (with the skin on) and squeeze out the excess moisture.

Put the coconut yogurt into a large mixing bowl and add the strained cucumber, garlic, dill, salt, pepper, lemon juice and maple syrup. Stir to combine.

Taste and adjust the flavour as needed. Serve immediately, or thicken in the refrigerator for 5 hours first.

ROAST CAULI WHITE BEAN DIP

Such an incredibly creamy yet healthy dip that's amazing served up on crusty sourdough. This dip is a great way to get kids to eat healthy veggies and beans without even realising it!

Serves 4

1 cauliflower, chopped
1 garlic clove
4 teaspoons olive oil, plus extra to garnish
½ teaspoon dried thyme
400g (14oz) can cannellini beans, drained
Juice of ½ lemon
Fresh parsley, to garnish (optional)
Salt and black pepper

Preheat the oven to 170°C/340°F/gas mark 3.

Place the cauliflower and garlic on a baking tray. Drizzle with 1 teaspoon of the olive oil and season with sea salt, black pepper and thyme. Roast the cauliflower for 20–25 minutes, or until browned, then allow to cool, discarding the garlic.

In a food processor, add the cauliflower, cannellini beans, lemon juice and remaining olive oil. Process for 3–5 minutes, or until the mixture is smooth. Adjust seasonings to taste. Garnish with a drizzle of olive oil and the parsley, if using.

CARROT AND CUMIN MISO BUTTER

Lovely melted on asparagus, broccoli or a baked sweet potato, this delicious dip pairs the natural sweetness of carrots with the deep, earthy flavour of miso. If you're fed up of regular hummus or yogurt dips, this is a tasty, unusual alternative.

Serves 4

400g (14oz) carrots, peeled and chopped
3 tablespoons olive oil
2 garlic cloves
1 teaspoon ground cumin
½ teaspoon ground ginger
400g (14oz) can cannellini beans, drained
2 tablespoons miso paste
Juice of ½ lime
1 tablespoon sesame oil
Salt

TO GARNISH
Fresh coriander (cilantro), chopped
Sesame seeds
Cumin seeds

Put the carrots, olive oil, garlic, cumin, ginger and salt into a saucepan. Cover with a very low layer of water and gently boil for 20–30 minutes, or until the carrots are soft. Drain, but keep the water to one side as you may need to blend a little back in.

Stir the cannellini beans through the carrot mixture. Put the mixture into a food processor, add the miso paste, lime juice and sesame oil and blend until smooth. If the mixture is too thick, add a little of the cooking water to loosen it.

Garnish with fresh coriander (cilantro), sesame seeds and cumin seeds.

LOADED *nachos*

This is not a dip, but rather a celebration of several kinds of dip. Is there anything more satisfying than a loaded tray of piping hot nachos? Grab a large bag of tortilla chips, cover them in vegan grated cheese and heat on a baking tray at 180°C/350°F/gas mark 4 for about 5 minutes. Remove from the oven and load up with the following:

Serves 4–6

TOMATO-LESS SALSA

300ml (10fl oz) Tomato-less Sauce
   (see page 61)
½ red onion, finely chopped
2 garlic cloves, minced
Small splash white wine vinegar
Juice of ½ lime
1 tablespoon extra virgin olive oil
Handful of fresh coriander (cilantro),
   roughly chopped

Combine everything in a bowl. Stir, then refrigerate until ready to serve.

SOURED CASHEW CREAM

150g (5¼oz) cashews
Juice of ½ lemon
1 teaspoon apple cider vinegar
½ teaspoon Dijon mustard
½ teaspoon salt

Add the cashews to a blender cup, cover in boiling water and soak for 30 minutes.

Drain half the water. Add the lemon, apple cider vinegar, mustard and salt and blend until smooth. Place in the refrigerator to cool.

GUACAMOLE

2 ripe avocados
½ small red onion, finely chopped
Juice of ½ lime
Pinch of salt
Large handful of fresh coriander (cilantro), chopped

Pit the avocados and scoop the flesh into a bowl. Mash the avocado with the back of a fork.

Add the onion, lime juice and a pinch of salt, then stir through well. Add the fresh coriander (cilantro) and stir in.

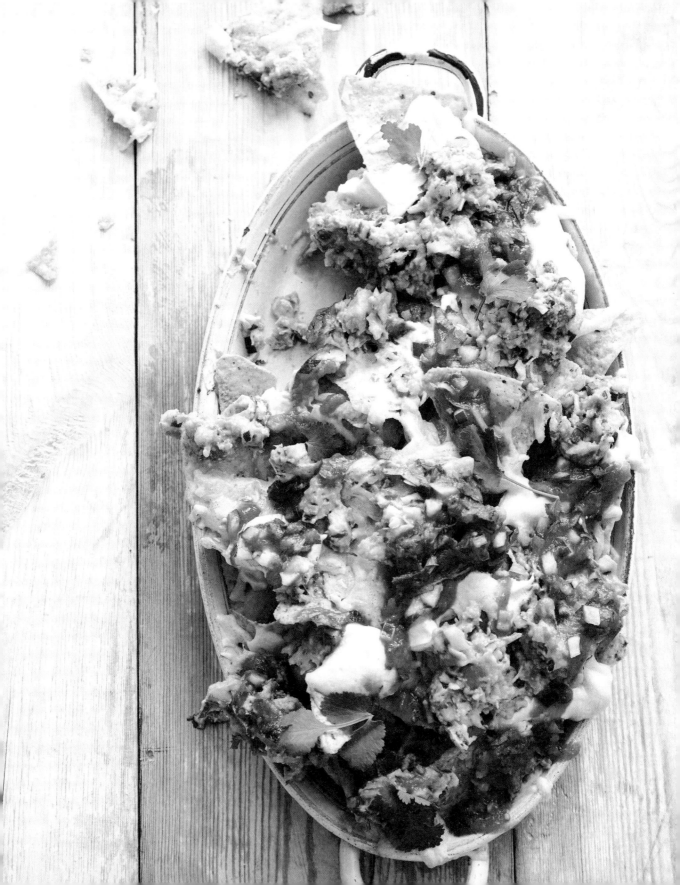

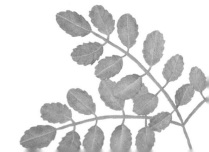

{ fermented }

FERMENTED FOODS

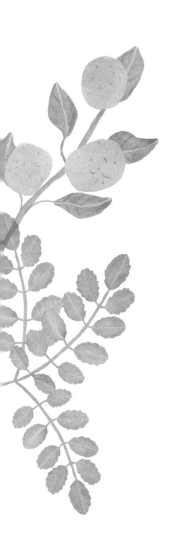

Fermented foods, such as sauerkraut, miso and kombucha are increasing in popularity thanks to their gut-friendly benefits. I wrote at the beginning of this book about the importance of gut health and its massive impact on this skin-healing journey. The key to working on good skin health is to begin replenishing the plethora of good bacteria that live in our gut, and the fastest way to do this is by consuming probiotics. Through the process of fermenting foods, the good bacteria grow, and these probiotics are transferred to our gut during digestion.

You might have seen jars of sauerkraut that you can buy off the shelf at the supermarket. Unfortunately, these are mostly pickled with vinegar and not with the natural fermentation process, which use live organisms. This means they don't contain probiotics. That's not to say prepackaged sauerkraut is necessarily bad for you, it just means you're not getting anywhere near as many benefits from the shop-bought stuff as you would from making your own.

Organic and whole-food health stores do sometimes sell the real deal. To ensure the fermented foods you buy do actually contain probiotics, look for the words "naturally fermented" on the label. When you open the jar, telltale bubbles in the liquid should signal that live organisms are present. If you're still uncertain, your safest bet is to make your own.

The fermenting process was new to me this year: I invited a lovely lady called Janice Clyne to join me on my podcast, and it's Janice who convinced me to get started. Janice is a highly qualified food scientist

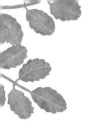
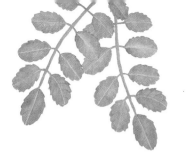

who ditched the corporate food world, and now spends her time sharing fermentation recipes at her little Scottish workshops. She is a self-confessed fermenting obsessive and has even had to buy an extra fridge to accommodate her ferments! It's difficult to speak to Janice and not get excited about the simple action of soaking vegetables in brine. Such an easy thing to do, and yet it offers a massive number of benefits.

GET PREPPED

Starting your first ferment is so easy! Yes, you can buy special preserving pots, but I always have so many glass jars knocking around from buying coconut oil, olives, mustard, artichoke hearts and more, so reusing these is a great way of cutting down on waste. You'll need wide-mouth jars to pack in all the ingredients, and it's really important to sterilize your jars before you begin (see note below).

Fermenting is actually super easy. It felt so daunting when I first began, but there really aren't many rules to successful fermentation. Ensuring your vegetables are well covered by brine is perhaps the most important. It's also key to use filtered water, as the chlorine in our tap water can stop the fermentation process in its tracks. And rather than regular table salt, use an alkaline option that is full of minerals, such as pink Himalayan salt.

Note: To sterilize your jars, wash them in hot, soapy water, rinse, then place in a preheated oven at 140°C/275°F/gas mark 1 to dry completely.

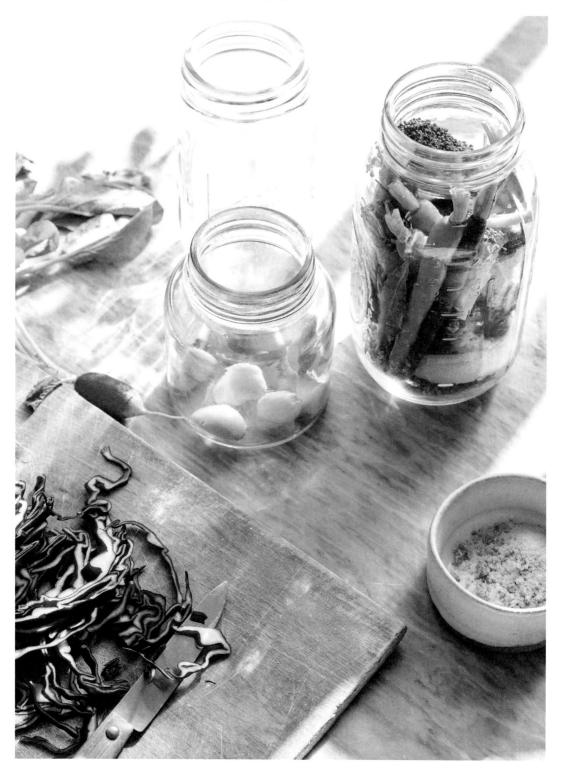

FERMENTED
garlic cloves

I'm a big garlic lover, but even I find the taste of raw garlic pretty intense. Recipes such as pesto or hummus, for example, taste that little bit more mellow when made with fermented garlic and it's a fantastic ingredient to use to add probiotics to salads or on top of pizza.

If you struggle with strep throat, fermented garlic is a brilliant antifungal, antibacterial and anti-inflammatory food that will help prevent the infection taking hold. This is a favourite recipe of mine because it's so easy to make. All it requires is a little patience.

Makes 1 1-litre (1¾-pint) jar

2 large bulbs of garlic
1 tablespoon pink Himalayan salt
1 litre (1¾ pints) filtered water

Peel each clove and pop them a sterilized 1-litre (1¾-pint) jar. Create a salt brine by dissolving the salt in the water.

Add the brine to the jar to cover the garlic. Ensure they're fully submerged in the brine (you might need to add a little weight, such as smaller, sterilized jar filled with brine, to ensure they stay under the water). Put the lid on the jar and set it on your kitchen counter out of direct sunlight.

Open the jar daily to release the pressure created by fermentation. As you do this, there should be a strong smell of garlic, especially once the fermentation really gets going.

It might take up to a week for the fermentation to begin. You can tell when you see tiny bubbles in the brine. After a while, the brine will take on a lovely golden-brown colour.

Let the garlic continue to ferment for at least a month for best results, but you can leave it longer if you wish. When you decide that it is done, screw the lid on firmly and store in the refrigerator.

RED CABBAGE *sauerkraut*

This recipe not only tastes delicious thanks to the addition of those magical little caraway seeds, it's also a great food source of L-Glutamine (see page 117) due to the deep fermentation processes that create an abundance of enzymes and good bacteria. This in turn allows amino acids and other nutrients to be better absorbed

Makes 1 1-litre (1¾-pint) jar

1 medium red cabbage
1 tablespoon pink Himalayan salt
1 litre (1¾ pints) filtered water
1 teaspoon caraway seeds (optional)

Rinse the cabbage in cool water. Remove the coarse outer leaves and discard. Remove and rinse a few unblemished leaves and set them aside. Rinse the cabbage again in cool water and place on a cutting board.

Using a large, sharp knife, slice the cabbage thinly. Place in a mixing bowl and massage the salt into the cabbage for 5 minutes, rest for 5 minutes, then repeat. You should end up with a much-reduced volume of cabbage sitting in its own brine in the mixing bowl.

Mix in the caraway seeds, if using. Now begin stuffing the cabbage very tightly into a sterilized 1-litre (1¾-pint) glass jar. Pour any excess liquid from the bowl into the jar. Ensure the brine covers the cabbage entirely – if needed, you can use one of the reserved leaves from earlier to push everything down under the brine. Loosely screw on a lid.

Fermentation will begin within a day and take 1–3 weeks depending on temperature and desired flavour. After a week, taste the sauerkraut. Technically, it will be slightly fermented after only a few days, but the best flavour seems to be at about the two- or three-week mark. Once fermented, it can be eaten right away, or stored in the refrigerator for up to six months.

> **NOTE:**
> It is normal to see bubbles, white scum or foam on top during the fermentation. You should not see any mould – if you do, you need to discard your sauerkraut and start again.

FERMENTED
vegetables

Fermented vegetables are a great and tasty way to get a daily dose of probiotics to maintain gut health. While you can ferment pretty much any vegetable you wish, you'll want to make sure the ingredients in your jar are roughly the same shape and size. This will ensure that they all ferment at the same rate.

Makes 1 1-litre (1¾-pint) jar

2–3 tablespoons salt
1 litre (1¾ pints) filtered water
Bunch of radishes
4 broccoli florets
2 carrots
1 tablespoon mustard seeds
¼ lemon
1 bay leaf
cabbage leaves (optional)

Completely dissolve the salt in 1 litre (1¾ pints) of filtered water.

Wash the radishes well and cut into quarters, then wash and slice the carrots and cut the broccoli into small florets.

Place the mustard seeds, lemon and bay leaf at the bottom of a sterilized 1-litre (1¾-pint) glass jar. Pack the vegetables on top.

Pour the salt water over the vegetables until it reaches just below the top of the jar. There should be about 1.25cm (½ inch) of room left. Ensure the vegetables are fully submerged; you might want to use a cabbage leaf to keep everything below the water line.

Close the lid on the jar tightly and place the jars out of direct sunlight at room temperature. You will start to see some bubbling on day two. Carefully unscrew the lid daily to release excess pressure.

The vegetables will be ready anywhere from day four to day ten. The longer they sit, the tangier they will become. Once ready, transfer to the refrigerator where they'll keep for a couple of months. These are great on salads or as a sandwich filler.

{ sweet }

BAKED LEMON CHEESECAKE
with fresh raspberries

Cheesecakes have always been one of my favourite desserts. While raw vegan cheesecakes are lovely in their own right, they never quite taste as indulgent as those rich, creamy, New York bakery-style ones – and that's what I wanted to recreate here.

Serves 8

FOR THE BASE
- 150g (5½oz) blanched almonds
- 100g (3½oz) porridge oats
- Pinch of salt
- 4 tablespoons coconut oil, melted
- 2 tablespoons maple syrup

FOR THE CHEESECAKE FILLING
- 200g (7oz) cashews (soaked for 1 hour in boiling water, then drained)
- 160ml (5½fl oz) coconut cream
- 170g (6oz) vegan cream cheese
- 1 teaspoon vanilla extract
- Juice and zest of ½ lemon, plus more zest to decorate
- 4 tablespoons maple syrup (or more if you like it really sweet)
- 1 tablespoon coconut oil
- Pinch of salt
- 200g (7oz) fresh raspberries, to decorate

Preheat the oven to 160°C/325°F/gas mark 3.

Add the base ingredients to a food processor and pulse until combined. They should form a doughy texture that you can shape with your hands. Press into a 20cm (8-inch) springform cake tin and bake for 15 minutes. Allow to cool, leaving the oven on.

Meanwhile, blitz the filling ingredients (except the raspberries) in a high-speed blender until completely smooth. Pour this mixture over the base and return to the oven for 45 minutes. Check to see if the edges are firm. They may brown a little, and the centre will still have some "give" in it, but it should not be liquid.

Remove from the oven and let cool for ten minutes before transferring to the refrigerator and leaving it to set for a couple of hours or overnight. Decorate with fresh raspberries and lemon zest to serve.

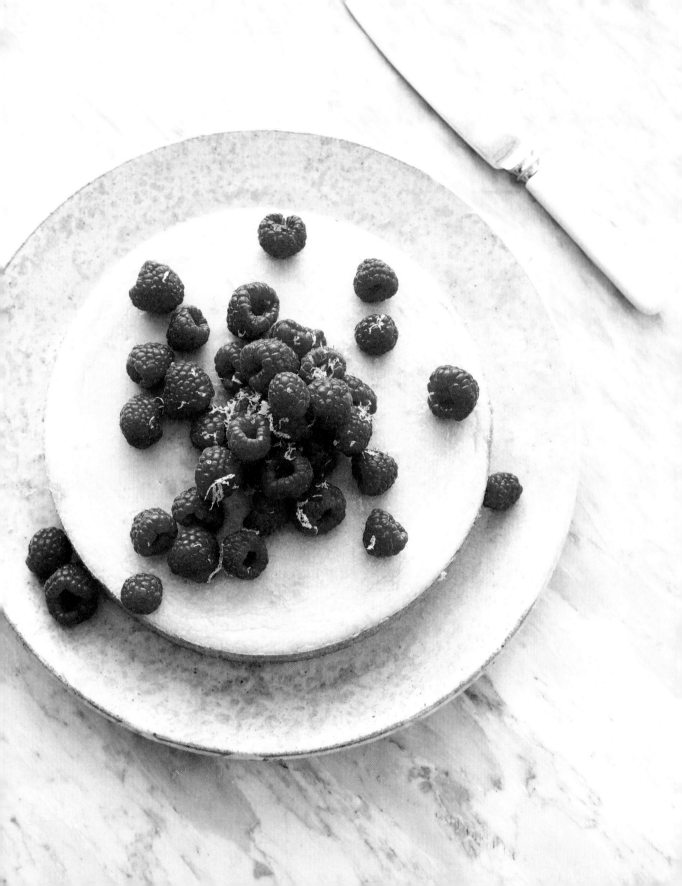

VEGAN *blondies*

I love this extra-easy and adaptable blondie recipe. These decadent, American-style dessert bars are the fairer cousin of the brownie, with the same dense and fudgy texture. The blondies taste like deep, rich, buttery caramel. If you're more partial to a brownie, you can simply add in some cacao powder to transform the recipe.

Makes 9

2 × 400g (14oz) cans chickpeas, drained
200g (7oz) gluten-free oats
1 teaspoon vanilla extract
75g (2¾oz) coconut sugar
2 tablespoons maple syrup
½ teaspoon baking powder
2 heaped tablespoons almond butter
1 tablespoon coconut oil
2 pinches of pink Himalayan salt

Preheat the oven to 180°C/350°F/gas mark 4.

Blend all the ingredients together on a slow setting in a food processor until smooth and well combined.

Pour into a 20cm (8 inch) square silicone baking tray or a metal baking tray lined with greaseproof paper. Bake for 30 minutes.

Stand to cool, then pop in the refrigerator to set for 1–2 hours. Slice into squares and store in the refrigerator.

You'd never know these rich, decadent treats are made with chickpeas!

PINEAPPLE
polenta cake

This gluten-free cake owes it pleasing texture to nuts, polenta and coconut, and its gentle tang to fresh pineapple. It's zingy, zesty and makes a wonderful pudding or afternoon tea.

Serves 6–8

130g (4½oz) polenta
100g (3½oz) ground almonds
150g (5½oz) self-raising flour (I use gluten-free)
½ teaspoon baking powder
150ml (5fl oz) almond or coconut yogurt
100ml (3½fl oz) coconut oil, melted
100ml (3½fl oz) maple syrup
75ml (2½fl oz) pineapple juice (the juice from a can of chunks works well)

Stir the polenta, ground almonds, flour and baking powder together.

In a separate mixing bowl, whisk together the yogurt, coconut oil, maple syrup and pineapple juice. Add the dry ingredients and whisk again.

Pour the mixture into a silicone loaf tin and bake for 45 minutes. Check the cake: you should be able to insert a skewer and it will come out clean. Pop the cake back in the oven if it needs a little longer.

When the cake is done, pour over a little more maple syrup and pineapple juice while it cools if you want it extra moist.

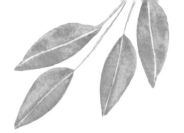

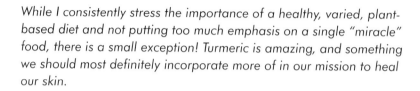

TURMERIC

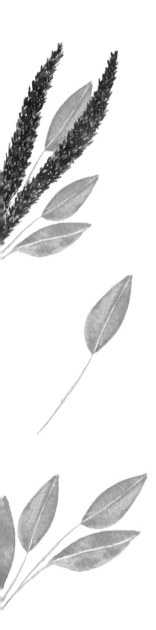

While I consistently stress the importance of a healthy, varied, plant-based diet and not putting too much emphasis on a single "miracle" food, there is a small exception! Turmeric is amazing, and something we should most definitely incorporate more of in our mission to heal our skin.

You've probably heard a great deal about this awesome spice. It has become increasingly popular over the past few years. But why is it so good for us? Firstly, we should consider its anti-inflammatory and antibacterial benefits: turmeric can work wonders by reducing redness from blemishes and calming conditions such as eczema and rosacea. Turmeric is excellent for acne because it is a natural antiseptic, which helps to keep bacteria from spreading.

When it comes to autoimmune conditions, curcumin – the active component in turmeric – is a fantastic immune system modulator. Rather than suppressing our immune system response, turmeric helps to get it back in balance. This makes it particularly powerful in supporting a psoriasis-healing protocol. Turmeric also stimulates the enzymes responsible for flushing out toxins, which makes it an effective liver protector (see page 121).

Ground turmeric can have a pungent, bitter flavour with hints of orange and ginger. It loses some of its essential oils and pungency in the drying process, but it can still provide warmth and colour to any dish. Fresh turmeric can be found in the produce section of larger grocery stores, health food shops and Asian or Indian supermarkets. It looks a little bit like root ginger, although its flesh is a much brighter orange colour. Be careful when cooking with turmeric: its bright, beautiful colour will stain pretty much everything it touches, and it's not easy to wash out!

On the page opposite you'll find two of my favourite recipes for cooking with turmeric. I've always loved cookies – in fact, when I was little, my nickname was "*Koekie*", Dutch for "cookie", as my mother is from Holland. These turmeric and ginger cookies are not only delicious, they also come with skin-healthy benefits. And while we're on a turmeric roll, my spiced turmeric latte is a great way to step away from caffeinated drinks in favour of a soothing, delicious latte infused with anti-inflammatory properties, meaning it is as good for you as it is tasty.

TURMERIC *& ginger cookies*

Makes 10

- 200g (7oz) jumbo oats
- 100g (3½oz) plain flour (I use gluten-free)
- 75ml (2½fl oz) maple syrup
- 1 teaspoon vanilla extract
- 100ml (3½fl oz) coconut oil, melted
- Pinch of salt
- 1 teaspoon baking powder
- 1 teaspoon ground turmeric (more if you love the taste)
- 1 teaspoon ground ginger (more if you love the taste)
- Handful of dried apricots, chopped

Preheat the oven to 170°C/340°F/gas mark 3. Line a baking tray with greaseproof paper.

Combine all the ingredients together well in a mixing bowl. Pick up a handful of the mixture and roll into a ball. Squish the ball flat and form into a thick cookie shape. Place the cookies on the lined baking tray. Bake for just 10–15 minutes.

The cookies will come out all soft and crumbly so don't touch them! Let them fully cool as they'll carry on baking a little in the tray. These will keep in an airtight tin for up to a week.

SPICED TURMERIC *latte*

Serves 2

- 300ml (10fl oz) coconut, oat or almond milk
- 1 teaspoon ground turmeric
- ½ teaspoon ground cinnamon, plus extra for sprinkling
- Pinch of ground ginger
- 1 teaspoon vanilla extract
- 2 teaspoons maple syrup
- Pinch of black pepper
- Pinch of salt

Warm the coconut or almond milk in a saucepan over a low heat for 5 minutes.

Whisk in the spices, vanilla, maple syrup, salt and black pepper. Pour carefully into two mugs and sprinkle with extra cinnamon.

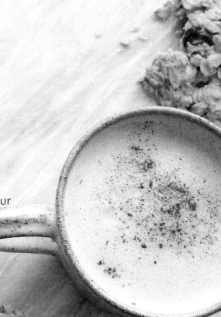

CHOCOLATE
mud cake

Decadent, rich and excessive, this is the ultimate vegan chocolate mud cake. Topped with a smooth, creamy and healthy chocolate mousse and fresh coconut yogurt, this makes the perfect centrepiece at any celebration.

Serves 6–8

375g (13oz) gluten-free self-raising flour
25g (1oz) raw cacao powder
400ml (14fl oz) almond milk
100g (3½oz) coconut sugar
150ml (5fl oz) light olive oil
2 teaspoons baking powder
1 tablespoon vanilla extract

FOR THE CHOCOLATE TOPPING
1 avocado (ripe or a little over ripe),
    peeled and pitted
2 tablespoons maple syrup (or more,
    if you like it sweet)
2 tablespoons cacao powder,
    plus extra for dusting
Drop of almond milk
100g (3½oz) coconut yogurt

Preheat the oven to 170°C/340°F/gas mark 3. Grease a 20cm (8 inch) spring-form cake tin.

Add the flour, cacao, almond milk, sugar, olive oil, baking powder and vanilla extract to a large mixing bowl and blend together well.

Pour into the cake tin and pop into the oven. Bake for 25–35 minutes.

Meanwhile, make the topping by blitzing all the ingredients except the coconut yogurt in the blender until smooth.

Skewer the cake to check it's baked. Leave a little longer if needed. Remove from the oven and allow to cool.

Serve topped with the chocolate cream and coconut yogurt, dusted with a little cacao powder.

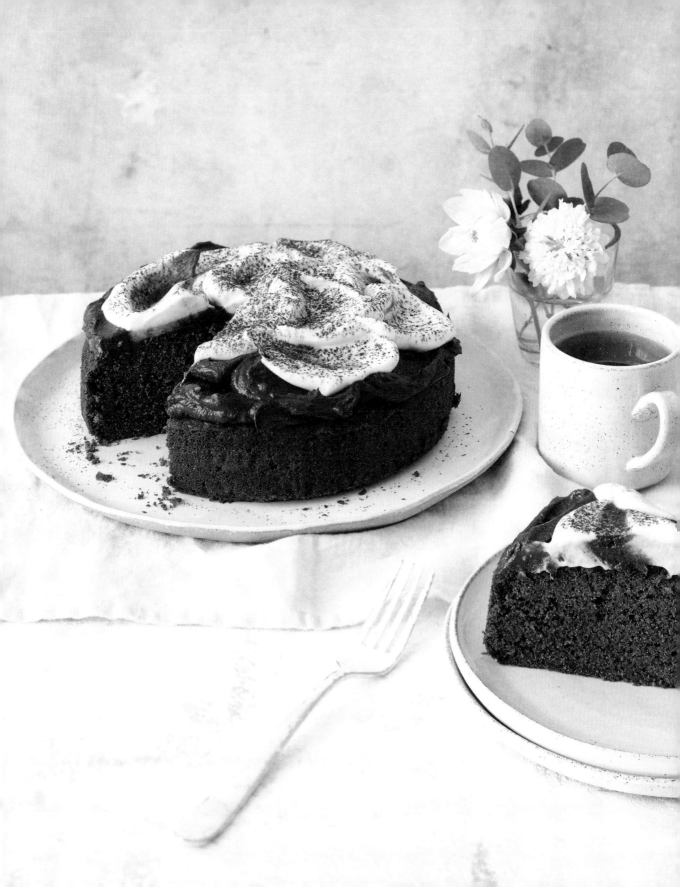

BLUEBERRY &
coconut panna cotta

This blueberry coconut panna cotta is quick to throw together, but it's so pretty it's sure to impress your friends. Sweet, creamy and yummy, this will definitely become one of your favourite go-to dinner party desserts.

Makes 3

400ml (14fl-oz) can coconut milk
1 tablespoon maple syrup
1 heaped teaspoon agar agar powder
100g (3½oz) frozen blueberries

Bring the coconut milk to the boil in a pan and stir in the maple syrup and agar agar. Reduce the heat to a simmer and keep whisking everything for 2–3 minutes.

Strain the liquid to remove any lumps, then pour into three 125ml (4fl oz) jelly moulds. Pop in the refrigerator for 2 hours, or until set.

Warm the frozen blueberries over a low heat for 5 minutes, and pour over to serve.

This will become one of your favourite go-to dinner party desserts

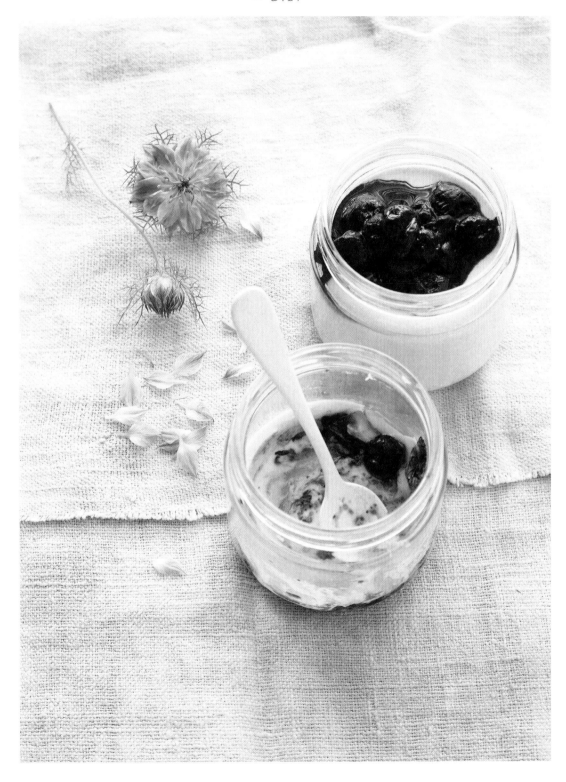

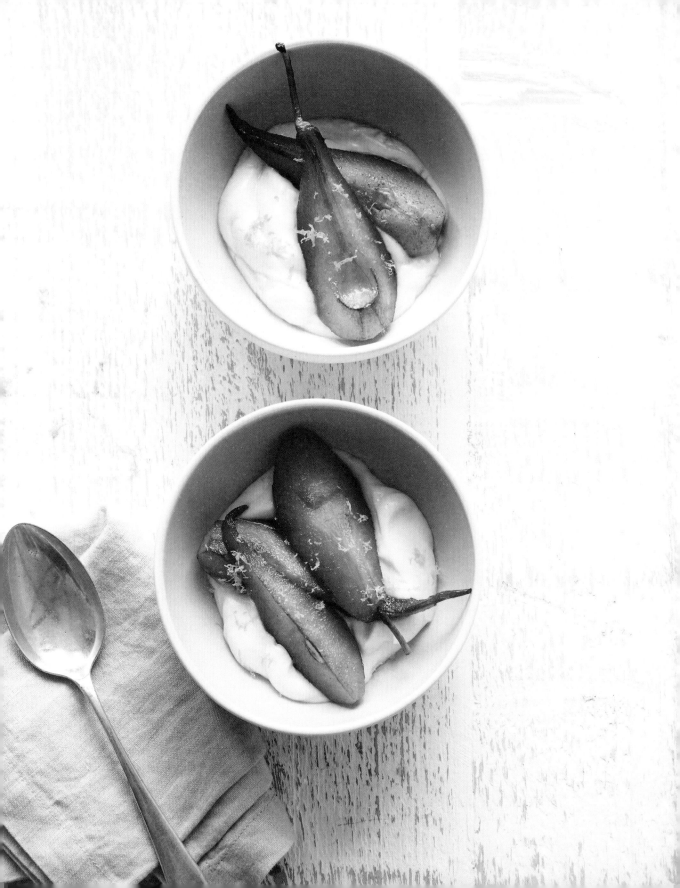

POMEGRANATE
poached pears

Sometimes a dessert doesn't have to be excessively rich and indulgent to be delicious. These wonderfully light poached pears look so elegant and taste amazing. They're easy to make and the combination of sweet and zesty flavours is just perfect.

Serves 2

1 tablespoon coconut oil
3 firm pears, peeled, halved and cored
300ml (10fl oz) pomegranate juice
100ml (3½fl oz) plus 1 teaspoon maple syrup
1 tablespoon vanilla extract
1 cinnamon stick
150g (5½oz) coconut yogurt
2 teaspoons lemon zest, to decorate

Melt the coconut oil in a frying pan over a medium heat. Add the pears, cut-side down, and cook until browned, about 5 minutes.

Add the pomegranate juice, 100ml (3½fl oz) of maple syrup, vanilla extract and cinnamon stick. Simmer gently until the pears are tender when pierced with the tip of a sharp knife, about 20 minutes. Turn very gently once or twice as they cook so they colour evenly.

Using a slotted spoon, transfer the pears to a shallow bowl and set aside. Let them cool slightly.

Stir together the coconut yogurt and remaining teaspoon of maple syrup in a small bowl. Spoon over the pears and decorate with lemon zest.

SUPPLEMENTS

Sourcing our nutrients from foods is my absolute preferred way to ensure we're getting all the vitamins and nourishment we need. Our bodies absorb these nutrients much better as part of a complex, whole food, but there are most definitely occasions when, due to additional life pressures such as a change in environment, working abroad, a vacation or other factors, we simply can't eat as good a variety as we would like. At these times, using good-quality supplements can be an excellent way to ensure you're still getting all the vitamins you need to support your skin-healing protocol.

PROBIOTICS

Since we're talking about good gut health, it's important to mention a supplement I recommend to anyone working to build a healthy digestive tract – probiotics. Probiotics are designed to help restore the natural balance of bacteria in your gut, particularly when it has been disrupted by an illness, medication or longstanding poor diet.

Our gut contains billions of bacteria from over 500 different species, all of which, when in balance, contribute to a healthy digestive system, metabolism and good hormonal health. These flora act as a sort of barrier against any harmful bacteria that may enter, and probiotics (also known as "good bacteria") help them to keep everything in check.

You can get healthy doses of probiotics from fermented foods such as sauerkraut, kimchi, kombucha or miso (see page 98), but if you're not able to consume these regularly, one of the best ways to boost your probiotic intake is through taking a supplement.

Research shows that some strains seem to be more effective than others for treating certain conditions. For example, the strains *Lactobacillus*, *L. acidophilus*, and *B. bifudum* have been found to be particularly effective in treating acne.

VITAMIN D

If you struggle with an autoimmune skin disease such as psoriasis, you might notice that exposure to sunlight improves your condition. Speaking personally, spending time in the sun always helps my skin to look and feel healthy. Our bodies manufacture vitamin D upon exposure to sunshine, but the level in many countries is so weak during the winter months that our body makes little to none at all.

The sun's UVB rays are effective at treating psoriasis symptoms because they slow the rapid rate of skin growth and shedding, but vitamin D also plays an integral role in skin protection and rejuvenation. In its active form as calcitriol, vitamin D contributes to skin cell growth, skin cell repair and metabolism. Functionally speaking, vitamin D more closely resembles a hormone than a vitamin. It optimizes the skin's natural immune system and helps destroy free radicals that can cause premature ageing.

A study published in the *British Journal of Dermatology* in 2011 found that people with psoriasis tend to have low vitamin D levels, particularly in colder seasons. Gradual exposure to sunlight can be particularly helpful, and if I'm in a climate where I know I'm going to struggle to maintain adequate levels, I ensure I regularly take a vitamin D supplement throughout those colder months.

CBD

Cannabidiol, more commonly referred to as CBD oil, is breaking new grounds in the healthcare industry. Promoted as a cure for everything from chronic pain to depression, arthritis and skin disease, you'd be forgiven for thinking this is a one-stop, cure-all miracle oil. Unsurprisingly, CBD oil has been receiving massive attention in recent years, given all these potential health benefits.

According to the National Eczema Association (NEA): "It has long been observed that cannabinoids possess anti-inflammatory, antimicrobial and anti-itch qualities" with research dating back to the first textbook of dermatology referencing a use for cannabis in treating skin conditions. Because of these powerful antioxidant and anti-inflammatory properties, CBD oil is thought to decrease the redness, itching and inflammation associated with many skin conditions. It can also help inhibit excessive oil secretion, which is one of the principal causes of acne. When it comes to psoriasis, CBD oil has been shown to decelerate skin cell division as cannabinoids

help normalize the cycle, leading to the reduction of scaly skin.

L-GLUTAMINE

You might have seen this in vitamin and health food stores, often marketed to athletes as a great way to repair muscle tissue. Science is now showing that glutamine benefits are abundant: It promotes digestive and brain health and boosts athletic performance, plus this amino acid is especially helpful in treating leaky gut and improving overall health. It's a simple and inexpensive supplement, and yet it can have a profound impact on gut health.

Glutamine is one of twenty naturally occurring amino acids in dietary protein. Because glutamine is the major fuel source for cells of the small intestine, it has been shown to heal leaky gut in clinical studies. Leaky gut is when your gut lining is too permeable – meaning things that shouldn't flow through your gut lining and into your bloodstream, do. L-Glutamine is all about feeding your gut with the fuel it needs to strengthen to stop this happening. When the gut barrier strengthens, the inflammation in your body begins to slow down since fewer and fewer toxins are successfully hitting your bloodstream.

If you find yourself constantly craving sugar, or struggling to quit alcohol, you might also find taking L-Glutamine useful. It has been found to help reduce, and even eliminate, cravings by helping to steady blood sugar levels. L-Glutamine is best taken with cold or room temperature water, so it's good to take in between meals on an empty stomach.

Using good-quality supplements can support your skin-healing protocol

Although there are rarely any negative side effects, if you are taking oral glutamine long-term, it's a good idea to also supplement with B vitamins, especially B12, which regulates glutamine build up in the body.

Red cabbage is an abundant plant-based source. Eating cabbage in the form of sauerkraut will increase its gut healing abilities, since the fermentation provides your gut with probiotics that also help make L-Glutamine more bioavailable (see page 116). Here are some more food-based sources:

- apricots
- asparagus
- beans
- beets
- broccoli
- cabbage
- lentils
- nuts
- peas
- prunes
- spinach
- tofu
- watercress

VITAMIN B12

B12 is mainly found in meat, eggs and dairy products. It is the only vitamin that is not recognized as being reliably supplied from a varied whole-food, plant-based diet with plenty of fruit and vegetables, together with exposure to sunshine. While seaweed, algae and certain mushrooms all contain vitamin B12, they are not reliable sources because they do not act the same way in the human body. There are however some vegan foods that are fortified with vitamin B12. These include non-dairy milks, nutritional yeast and veggie spreads such as Marmite.

Typical deficiency symptoms include loss of energy, tingling, numbness, reduced sensitivity to pain or pressure, blurred vision, abnormal gait, sore tongue, poor memory, confusion, hallucinations and personality changes. Often these symptoms develop gradually over several months to a year before being recognized as being due to B12 deficiency.

Taking a B12 supplement is particularly important if you're planning to add L-Glutamine into your regime, as it regulates glutamine build up in the body.

In choosing to use fortified foods or B12 supplements, we vegans are taking our B12 from the same source as every other animal on the planet – microorganisms – without causing suffering to any sentient being or causing environmental damage.

ADDITIONAL VITAMINS

It can feel like a mammoth – not to mention expensive – addition to your daily routine, remembering to take a long list of supplements. If you know this is something you're going to struggle with, take a look through the recommendations and consider which ones are most important to you and which you might be able to source through making changes to your diet. Or, as with other parts of the plan, build vitamins into your routine gradually. Most supplements are not designed to be taken for the rest of your life, but to offer additional support while your body is healing or when you're struggling to source sufficient quantities naturally for whatever reason. To make things easier, look for a combined daily formula for skin, hair and nails, which will generally contain the vitamins I'd most highly recommend.

Consider which vitamins you might be able to source through your diet

VITAMIN E

Vitamin E helps support the immune system, cell function and skin health. It's an antioxidant, making it effective at combatting the effects of free radicals produced by the metabolism of food and toxins in the environment. Sunflower seeds, avocado and butternut squash are all good natural food sources.

RIBOFLAVIN B2

Riboflavin plays an important role in the repair of tissues, the healing of wounds and other injuries that can take a long time to fully recover. It helps to improve the skin's mucus secretion and might clean up the skin pustules that are common with acne. In the gut, riboflavin plays a major role in maintaining and protecting the mucous membranes in the digestive system. Good food-based sources include edamame beans, broccoli, asparagus, spinach and wild rice.

NIACIN

Also known as vitamin B3, niacin is an important nutrient. Every part of your body needs it to function properly. As a supplement, niacin aids in the normal functioning of the human digestive system, promoting a healthy appetite, properly functioning nerves and glowing skin. Avocado, mushrooms and leafy greens are all good plant-based sources.

SELENIUM

Selenium neutralizes free radicals and other skin-damaging compounds before they can lead to wrinkles. It's similar to vitamin E and actually works with that vitamin to safeguard cell membranes, the protective coating around cells. That makes selenium a key player when it comes to slowing the signs of ageing. Brazil nuts are a fantastic source. Eating just three to five a day is enough to reach the recommended allowance.

ZINC

Zinc is especially beneficial for inflammatory skin conditions and related scarring. Chickpeas, lentils, beans, chia seeds and quinoa are all great plant-based sources.

BETA-CAROTENE

We need vitamin A for healthy skin and mucous membranes, our immune system and good eye health and vision. Vitamin A can be sourced from the food we eat, through beta-carotene, for example, or in supplement form. Carrots, sweet potato, dark leafy greens and apricots are all good food sources.

COPPER

Copper helps build collagen, which is important to maintain skin elasticity, so it's safe to say that copper can improve skin firmness and reduce wrinkles. Shiitake mushrooms, raw cacao and dried fruits are good sources of copper.

GRAPESEED EXTRACT

Grapeseed extract is made from the crushed seeds of grape plants. Grape seeds contain many powerful nutrients, all of which help towards giving you a healthier, more radiant and hydrated complexion. Widely used in natural cosmetics, grape seed extract can also be taken as a supplement.

MAKING DECISIONS ON MEDICATION

Lots of people come to me feeling frustrated because their doctor has suggested they need to continue using pharmaceutical medication to clear their skin, implying they can't begin to heal naturally. However, pharmaceutical and natural healing protocols can work really well side by side, and working on your diet and lifestyle can often help you to gradually wean off medication in the long run.

Whichever treatment path you follow, the decision is yours and yours alone. Sure, people can advise you and you should always seek expert help, but you should never feel forced or pressured into following a particular protocol – be that medicinal or otherwise. Take time to think about your choices, ask for support from your doctor, but stand firm and make it clear you're not seeking approval, you're simply ensuring you won't be putting your life in danger by pursuing the treatment choices you are making.

If your doctor is dismissive or unsympathetic toward your questions around diet and lifestyle, you might like to speak to a naturopath. Naturopathy is a system of healthcare that promotes the body's own self-healing mechanism. It uses natural therapies such as nutrition, herbal medicine, acupuncture, homeopathy, hydrotherapy, physical manipulations, colonic irrigation, fasting, exercise and others. When it comes to lifestyle changes, patients often feel better understood by a naturopath who can help support a natural healing protocol.

In terms of emollients, medicated shampoos and, particularly, steroids, continued usage alongside a natural protocol again comes down to making some very personal decisions. There is no right or wrong. I've seen so much damage done in terms of thinning of the skin through long-term steroid use; and the flare–remission cycle you can experience through systematically applying and then eliminating usage is unpleasant. If you're using medicated creams – especially steroids – at the moment, I'd recommend gradually weaning off them over quitting cold turkey. Topical steroid withdrawal is a horrible experience, and while it doesn't affect everyone, most of us see some level of flare up when we stop using the cream that's been suppressing our symptoms for so long. Slowly reducing usage over time is a much safer way to prevent that negative reaction on the skin.

ANTIBIOTICS

Over-the-counter painkillers and drugs used to treat acid reflux, diabetes and psychiatric conditions have all been linked to microbiome changes, but perhaps the most cited gut-altering drugs of all are antibiotics. While the development of antibiotics has lengthened our lifespans, excessive and inappropriate use of these drugs can have serious long-term consequences. While antibiotics are prescribed to kill harmful bacteria, they can't differentiate between the good and the bad. Even a short course of antibiotics may cause permanent changes to the community of friendly flora in our gut. This isn't to say we should refuse antibiotic treatment – sometimes it is necessary and essential. If your doctor has prescribed antibiotics, it's important to take them as directed. We should, however, take these drugs only when appropriate and simultaneously work on mitigating any negative side effects, for example through replenishing lost bacteria.

It isn't just our own medication we ought to worry about. Antibiotics fed to livestock can enter the food chain through meat and dairy consumption. There is real concern that agricultural antibiotic use is driving up levels of antibiotic resistance, leading to new "superbugs".

In addition, a considerable number of antibiotics are used in healthy animals to prevent infection or speed up growth. This is particularly the case in intensive farming, where animals are kept in confined conditions. If you still eat fish, I would highly recommend wild caught over farmed. Fish farms have a long history of dosing fish they are breeding and rearing with antibiotics, as well as using fungicides and other chemicals to prevent disease – not drugs we want to be absorbing secondhand.

LONG LIVE YOUR LIVER

Our liver is responsible for two dominant functions that greatly affect our skin health: digestion and detoxification. Think of your liver as the body's filter. It sieves everything we come into contact with: the air we breathe, the food we eat, the water we drink – in fact anything we put into, or on to, our bodies. The liver also protects us from harmful chemicals, poisons, toxins, poor nutrition and more. Overburdening the liver through drugs, alcohol and cigarettes is obviously going to add additional stress, but we live in an age where our basic air, water and food are more toxic than ever before. This heavy burden can cause the liver to become fatigued and congested. When this happens, our health begins to decline and that can show up on the surface of our skin.

The liver is the organ most impacted by excess stress, unhappiness and worry. If you are often irritable, get angry easily, have trouble unwinding from the day's activities, find it hard to reason or struggle to let things go, you might be experiencing a liver problem. Feeling these emotions chronically or excessively can lead to seriously imbalanced liver function.

It comes as no surprise that when the liver becomes overtired like this, it struggles to eliminate toxins. In this instance, other organs such as the kidneys and skin have to pick up the slack, resulting in all those impurities exiting our body via the epidermis. Naturally this process can greatly upset our skin, especially if we're already struggling with dry and sensitive skin conditions. Toxins can easily cause irritation, itchiness and even a dreaded flare.

Diet plays a big part, too. Excessive refined sugar can cause wild fluctuations in blood sugar and insulin levels, which can significantly affect our mood and mental health. They also deplete B vitamins from the body, which can affect the nervous system. Too much caffeine can create "toxic heat" in the liver, causing a rise in anger and anxiety. As a stimulant, caffeine can ultimately lead to adrenal exhaustion and depression. Through supporting the detoxification and functioning of the liver, we can experience hormonal balance, less inflammation, excellent digestion, greater immunity, cleaner blood, a calmer mind and radiant skin.

ADVICE FOR LIVER HEALTH

• Cruciferous vegetables such as broccoli, cauliflower, kale, cabbage, rocket (arugula) salad and radishes contain DIM (diindolylmethane), which promotes the detoxification of the liver, especially of excess hormones. Ensure you incorporate lots of these as often as possible into your diet.

• Sulphur-rich foods such as Brazil nuts, almonds, onions, garlic, peaches and apricots are potent detoxifiers that help the liver. Sulphur is also great for collagen production, which can help keep skin youthful.

• Antioxidant-rich foods like berries, beetroot, mushrooms and raw cacao can help fight oxidative stress often caused by toxins and inflammation.

• Botanical herbs such as milk thistle contain extraordinary amounts of SOD (superoxide dismutase) and other flavonoids that help promote liver detoxification.

• Take action by eliminating other toxic substances, especially the ones you put on your skin. Anything absorbed by your skin goes directly to your liver to be filtered. Switch to 100 per cent natural skincare or experiment by making your own (see pages 158–185).

• Sweating leads to lipolysis (breaking down fat cells), which will help the body release toxins that are stored in fat. Whether you exercise, sunbathe or sit in an infrared sauna, encouraging your body to sweat away toxins can support good liver health.

LIVER CLEANSE *tea*

Proper liver function is essential to overall health as your liver helps remove waste products, processes various nutrients and aids in the absorption of vitamins. My liver cleanse tea offers a harmonious blend of herbs traditionally used for maintaining a healthy liver and supporting our body's natural cleansing process.

Makes enough for 30 cups (1 month's supply)

10g (¹/₃oz) peppermint
10g (¹/₃oz) dandelion root
5g (¼oz) liquorice root
10g (¹/₃oz) centaury
10g (¹/₃oz) rooibos
10g (¹/₃oz) yarrow

Combine the ingredients in an airtight jar.

To brew the tea, steep 2 teaspoons of the tea blend in hot water for 3–5 minutes, pouring the water over the leaves to bring out the flavours.

Strain the tea leaves and enjoy your liver cleanse tea warm.

Peppermint – stimulates bile flow and relaxes bile ducts. The bile juice helps in breaking down fats and also reducing bad cholesterol. In turn, it improves liver functioning.

Dandelion root – studies suggest that polysaccharides in dandelion may be beneficial to liver function.

Liquorice root – can reduce liver injury by enhancing antioxidant and anti-inflammatory capacity.

Centaury – the bitter compounds found in centaury can help stimulate bile production, helping the liver flush away toxins with more speed and ease. It helps purify the blood and is an excellent tonic for the digestive system.

Rooibos – can help improve liver function and protect it against oxidative damage.

Yarrow – stimulates the liver's activity and provides balance when needed.

LIVER SUPPORT
essential oil blend

The oils in this blend are hepatic in nature, which means that they stimulate, strengthen and tone the liver, helping increase bile flow and detoxification. Others are a great gallbladder support or aid in lymph circulation, which also supports a healthy liver.

Makes 30ml (1fl oz)

3 drops chamomile essential oil
5 drops geranium essential oil
5 drops patchouli essential oil
5 drops rosemary essential oil
6 drops ginger essential oil
Carrier oil (such as sweet almond or fractionated coconut oil)

To make an effective liver support blend, combine the oils in a 30ml (1fl oz) amber dropper bottle. Fill the dropper bottle to the shoulder with the carrier oil.

Apply one dropper full of liver support blend under your right ribcage. You can spread it across your abdomen and the middle of your back as well.

Use upon waking and before bedtime for best results.

Chamomile essential oil – stimulates bile secretions and supports liver detox.
Geranium essential oil – aides the liver by expanding the liver's bile ducts, which helps with detox.
Patchouli essential oil – tones and strengthens the liver and stomach.
Rosemary essential oil – enhances bile flow and prevents toxic overload.
Ginger essential oil – helps reverse a fatty liver and stimulates liver secretions.

CELERY *juice*

When it comes to the concept of "food as medicine", we can sometimes begin to get fixated on a particular food, vitamin or drink to resolve our skin issues – much like we've become used to taking a very specific medication to cure an illness. In reality there is no one particular food that will cure skin disease. Concentrating on a varied, plant-based diet is the best way to ensure your body is getting a powerful combination of vitamins and antioxidants.

It might feel as though the celery juice or liver cleanse fad has infiltrated every form of social media over the past couple of years, and yes, it does have some very awesome benefits. Celery contains impressive amounts of vitamins C and K, as well as folate and potassium. It also contains flavones, antioxidant compounds that can stop specific reactions in the body that lead to chronic inflammation, in turn lowering our risk of chronic skin flares.

Celery also contains sodium cluster salts, which are toxic to bacteria – including streptococcus – in the liver and lymphatic system. Your liver's individual immune system relies on these sodium cluster salts. When they come into contact with viruses, they break down the pathogen's cell membrane, which eventually kills the bacteria, viruses or microorganisms that can cause a huge range of issues, from digestive problems to acne, eczema, psoriasis and urinary tract infections.

Juiced celery alone can be a bit of a, let's say, acquired taste! Adding other fruits and veggies, such as cucumbers and apples, can make it more palatable while you are getting used to the flavour.

Serves 1

Bunch of celery
½ cucumber
1 apple (or more, if you prefer your juice sweeter)
½ lemon
2.5cm (1 inch) piece of fresh root ginger
Ice, to serve

Wash everything well, then juice. Serve over ice.

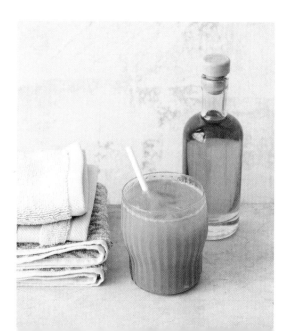

CASTOR OIL *pack*

The idea behind using a castor oil pack to treat the liver is to hold the oil on a piece of cloth against the skin for 45 minutes to 1 hour with a heat source to stimulate lymph and liver function. Unlike some "detox" methods, I find this gentle but effective, without any negative side effects. I also find it helps with better sleep, more energy and most importantly, clearing of skin symptoms. For the biggest benefits, I try to find a time when I can do this castor oil pack for three consecutive days. I'm always amazed at how much better I feel afterwards.

Makes 1 pack

Hot water bottle
2 old towels
A wash cloth
Castor oil

Find your liver: bring your fingers to the bottom of the right-side of your ribcage. The liver rests just under the very bottom of the ribcage, from the very right side of your body to the centre.

Prepare your hot water bottle and put one towel underneath you in a comfortable place. I usually do this in bed with a good book.

Place the wash cloth in a large glass dish (a large glass oven dish works well). Drizzle castor oil over the wash cloth until it's saturated, then place it over your liver. Cover your abdomen with the second towel and then place the hot water bottle on top.

Lie on your back with your feet slightly elevated (I usually lie on my bed with a pillow under my feet) and relax for 30–60 minutes.

Use a natural soap or a mix of bicarbonate of soda (baking soda) and water to remove any castor oil left on the skin. Or you can let it absorb into your skin.

Relax and rest. Ensure you drink enough water and stay hydrated after doing this to support your liver. You can keep the soaked cloth and re-use up to 10 times. Store in the refrigerator.

NOTES:
- Castor oil can stain, so wear old clothes and ensure you take care to place towels beneath you to protect the bedding.
- Ladies, avoid using a castor oil pack if you have an IUD because it could cause the IUD to dislodge or release excess copper. It's also not recommended when pregnant, breastfeeding, during your period or if you struggle with IBS, colitis or diarrhoea.

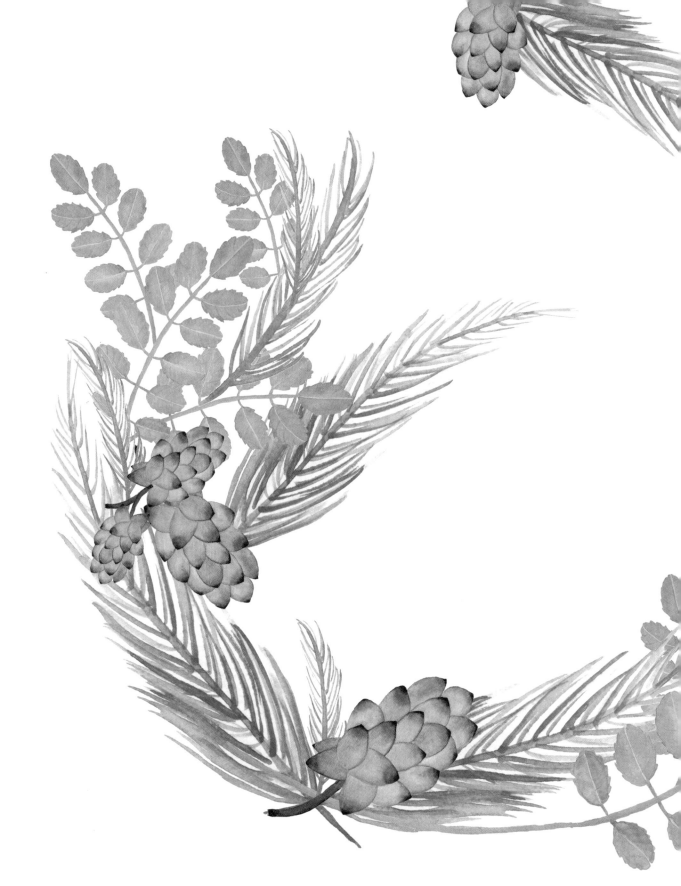

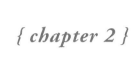

{ *chapter 2* }

mind

So many of us notice a correlation between a rise in stress levels and irritating skin flares. It can be a frustrating and vicious circle. When we get stressed, our skin seems to take it badly, then we become anxious as we see our skin getting worse, and that just exacerbates the problem. Our mind, gut and skin are so intrinsically connected, it's no wonder our skin seems to synchronize with our emotions. Mental health can be one of the more difficult aspects to tackle of this 5-pillar plan. Delving into the corners of our mind to deal with unresolved emotions can seem more daunting than adjusting our diet or exercising more regularly. I want to explain why I believe the brain to be an integral part of the healing jigsaw and to share with you my tips to begin calming your mind and, in turn, your skin.

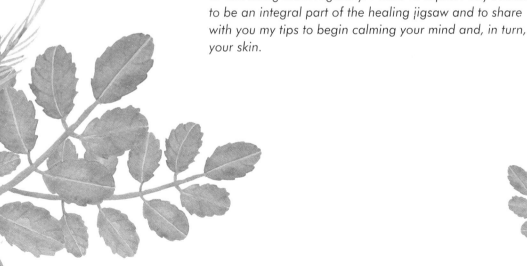

DANIELLE'S STORY

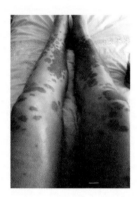 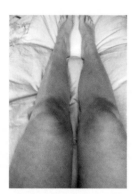

"I'd tried everything to treat my psoriasis, even resorting to three months of immunosuppressants. They didn't really offer a positive change and going for regular liver tests frightened me. I connected with Hanna on Instagram. Before then, I'd never thought about diet or lifestyle playing a role in my condition, but Hanna's pictures were amazing. I spoke excitedly to my dermatologist about dietary changes but she dismissed me. Instead of feeling disheartened, I used this negative response to empower me.

The online skin community is everything! I've learned so much about food and nutrition. As I started making changes, I saw results. It isn't a quick fix, but it's worth it. For me it isn't about instant healing. We all have the stressful roller coaster of life to manage and at times my skin is worse than others, but I finally feel I'm in control.

I'd let psoriasis control so much of my life, from the long-sleeved wedding dress I wore to not relaxing around the pool on my honeymoon. Now I try to encourage people to switch their mindset and wear the clothes they love. I'm a believer in 'fake it till you make it'! Stand tall, smile and strut your stuff. I practise gratitude everyday. My skin is amazing. It tells me when I'm stressed, it monitors my temperature, it protects my organs. I've learned to change my relationship with my skin and take back control. Your mind doesn't control you. Your skin doesn't control you. YOU are the boss!"

THE SKIN WARRIOR
power mindset

We live in a chaotic little world. When we're dealing with the exhaustion of chronic skin disease, we need every ounce of strength we can muster to battle the obstacles in our way and make life changes conducive to our health. A tenacious mind is essential. Being offered a chemotherapy drug when I was at rock bottom with my skin was a game changer for me. In that moment I had two choices: to curl up and quit, or to empower myself to make changes and get well again. It's that same mindset Danielle talked about opposite when her dermatologist dismissed her questions about the benefits of a natural healing programme. So, what gave Danielle the courage to go ahead?

A strong, empowered mind gives us an amazing capacity to face tough challenges head on. Being strong means having the resources, mental skills and physical capabilities to confront difficulties of all kinds through our battle with skin health. That true strength of character comes from a combination of mindfulness, focus and resilience. I find that strong-minded warriors such as Danielle have an amazing energy and stamina to face their healing challenge without being robbed of their inner strength. It's this mental dexterity that gives each of us the courage to grow from some of the most stressful situations we experience in life.

So, how do you achieve this miracle mindset? If you want a strong attitude, you can achieve it, but it's going to take work and patience. Just like growing muscles in a gym, you can develop your strength of character over time. You might connect with people on this skin-healing path who seem naturally mentally tougher than you are, or you might read Danielle's story thinking "I'm just not like that", but the good news is that you can learn to become equally strong. Having the conviction to live by your values, a willingness to learn and the resilience to recover from adversity are the key ingredients to achieving your power mindset.

SEEK HELP

In the same way as you might employ a personal trainer to help you exercise in the gym, working with a coach is such a great investment and support to improve your mental wellbeing. As with anything, strengthening your mind is something you can work at and achieve alone, but often the additional guidance that comes from a positive outside influence can be a fantastic starting point and ultimate game changer. So many of us feel unheard in our battle with skin disease, and there's something lovely about the simple act of being listened to again.

Do you feel there is still a stigma attached to seeking mental help? It's an odd one, isn't it? We might be quite open about working with a personal trainer or dietician to improve our body, but we're somehow embarrassed to admit we're seeking help for our mind. Going through important life challenges or difficult transitions can massively impact our ability to cope. This can affect how well we function and that, in turn, can impact our skin.

Think back to our circle of wellbeing (see page 8). Every choice we make can play a role in our skin health. Life's challenges include work-related stress, career problems, money worries, health concerns, family illness, the end of a relationship or close friendship and all sorts of decision-making challenges related to these testing times. Dealing with a skin condition on top of all this can be massive. You might feel as though your doctor or dermatologist hasn't listened or taken seriously your emotional wellbeing. Trying to cope with skin disease can add to a buildup of lots of these little problems, which eventually begin to feel like an overwhelming tidal wave.

Counselling can be super helpful in providing the support and skills to better

work through our most testing times. Rather than considering it embarrassing or thinking of yourself as somehow having failed, it's important to view this as an invaluable investment in your emotional, physical and mental health. It's an act of courage, not weakness. A positive gift to yourself and everyone around you.

GO IT ALONE

You might feel as though you're not ready to open up to anybody else about your problems just yet, or that it's a luxury you're unable to invest in due to financial constraints. If fear of the unknown is holding you back, just like that first session at the gym, it can be very tempting to skip it or run away. The big changes we want to see will only come about as a result of the big changes we're prepared to make. If seeking outside help is not an option right now, don't let that be an excuse not to do something.

I used to read lots of books about developing a positive mindset. I'd get really frustrated at anything that told me to monotonously repeat positive mantras or plaster sticky notes all over everything reminding me to "think happy thoughts"! Developing the right thoughts is not about being constantly upbeat or cheerful, and it isn't about ignoring anything negative or unpleasant in our lives. It's about embracing both the positives and negatives and still choosing to be generally optimistic. We can't all be 100 per cent happy 100 per cent of the time. It's okay to accept that this is normal and to embrace

Developing the right thoughts is about embracing both the positives and negatives

bad moods and difficult emotions when they arise, but speaking to ourselves in a much more positive, kinder way can really begin to change the way we think and feel.

We don't always have power over the thoughts that pop into our minds, but we can choose how we handle those thoughts and respond to them. When we give in to negativity, pessimism and a doom-and-gloom view of our wellbeing, we are not only submitting to a loss of control and potentially wallowing in unhappiness, we are also missing out on an important opportunity to learn something and grow from it.

LEARN TO DEAL WITH NEGATIVE THOUGHTS

Negative thoughts can pop up uninvited and leave behind a mess of tangled emotions. It's frustratingly easy to get stuck in the same old neural pathways, experiencing recurring negative thoughts like a broken record. We look down at our skin and hate what we see, that makes us feel helpless and out of control and the negative thought cycle perpetuates.

Our brains don't stop developing when we reach adulthood. Think about what happens when we master a new language or learn to play an instrument; our grey matter continually changes. There are incredible stories of neural pathways finding a way through, even after serious brain damage. Ultimately, we hold the power to stop these bad thoughts about our skin continually trampling down well-trodden neural pathways – by creating entirely new ones. You might have heard of something called CBT (cognitive behavioural therapy). Through CBT training, the brain learns to reinforce new positive neural pathways, so it becomes easier and easier to deal with future negative or stressful situations.

We all have an inner critic. I like to think of mine as a completely separate entity from myself. I can picture her, inside my head, ready to pop up at the most inconvenient moments to question me. In the privacy of my own mind she used to say things like "you can't wear that, your skin looks awful" or "find something with long sleeves, everyone is going to stare". I used to think that when this negative voice crept into my head, it was simply an extension of me, a perfectly normal part of who I am. But I've since come to realize my inner critic only ever focused on one specific way of looking at my skin (it was not a good one) when there were, in fact, many much more positive perspectives.

If a friend is asking us for advice on what to wear, we would never dream of speaking to them like our inner critic talks to us. Say they wanted to wear a strappy dress to a summer party and they had blotchy arms; we would never tell them "you shouldn't wear that, you will look awful, everyone will point at you". If that's our response, we're a pretty mean friend! So, why do we accept that it's okay to speak to ourselves like that? Think of somebody you admire for their strong mindset and imagine that person is standing beside you, offering support in relation to your skin. If they were rooting for you, what might they say?

Silencing your negative voice is about moving beyond the pessimistic chatter inside your head and putting that inner critic firmly back inside its box. Vow to be kinder to yourself, and begin that process by clearly defining your manifesto.

YOUR MANIFESTO

Your personal manifesto is a declaration of your values, beliefs and intentions when it comes to your wellbeing and this all important skin-healing journey.

Take some time to think about your personal manifesto. It will act as an inspiring reminder to focus on, and embrace, what's most important to you.

CAROLINE'S STORY

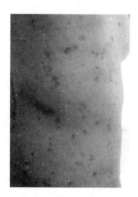 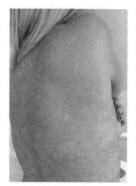

"My psoriasis started when I was thirty. I was covered in what looked like cigarette burns. I got a diagnosis and was put on UV treatment. More recently I struggled with an abusive relationship and a stressful job, and my skin flared badly. Scalp psoriasis really affected me and I was always conscious of flaking skin on my shoulders. My doctor suggested immunosuppressant drugs, which wasn't a route I wanted to go down.

I found Hanna's book, *Radiant,* a year ago. Athough I thought I was fairly healthy, I'd been eating lots of nightshades and dairy. I started following the plan and felt great. I managed to improve things, but I didn't always stick to it.

I realized I had to get out of my relationship and break my routine. I went on a month-long plant-based yoga retreat in Thailand. That respite from processed foods, caffeine, alcohol and sugar was a game changer. When I came home people didn't recognise me! Since then I've started teaching yoga three times a week. Exercise has been an important part of my healing. I'd had moments where I felt my skin was too bad to go to any exercise class, but yoga is open to anyone, at any age of any ability.

I still have scars from my psoriasis, but my scalp is clear. By following a good diet and making sure I take time to relax physically and mentally, I've broken free from the symptoms that plagued me for the past decade."

QUIET MIND
& meditation

Even though meditation has become much more commonplace over the past few years, the word itself can still conjure up mystical images of smoking incense and sitting in a circle, eyes closed, chanting a mantra in an Indian ashram.

In reality, meditation is far from intimidating and does not require you to be in any specific country or place of worship. Like doing anything new for the first time, it can feel a little strange or uncomfortable to begin with. But it's a simplistic tool that costs nothing and is open to all of us at any given moment. The most important thing we can do is begin to use it.

Meditation has been proven to help ease chronic pain, reduce anxiety, manage stress, improve heart health, boost mood and strengthen immunity. Research tells us that conditions caused or worsened by stress can be alleviated through meditating, and anecdotally so many of us struggling with skin conditions acknowledge that we see a very real correlation between heightened stress levels and skin flares.

Learning to meditate is not difficult, but like anything new it requires commitment and patience – which is why we call it a "practice". Meditation is a great way to increase awareness of yourself and your surroundings, in turn reducing stress and getting a healthy perspective on things. I always used to think that the purpose of meditation was switching off my thoughts or feelings, but rather than trying to make them disappear, it's about observing those thoughts without judgement.

My reluctance to get into meditation was based on the belief that I could be doing something more productive with my time! What was the point of sitting there in silence for ten minutes, when in reality I had work to finish or dinner to prepare? But meditation will actually make you *more* productive. It might sound strange that sitting still and doing nothing for a period of time will help you achieve more, but it's absolutely true.

When I first started to meditate, I remember being confused at what exactly I was supposed to do once I'd sat down. I was on a retreat in France and like a naughty school child I kept squinting through my eyes to check what everyone else was doing, in case I'd got it wrong! I felt so self-conscious.

The basic principle of meditation is simple. Set a short timer to begin with – two minutes is just fine. Sit still with your eyes closed and breathe. Every time your mind begins to shift its focus away from your breath and you get lost in thought, bring your attention back to the breath. Repeat this again and again until your meditation timer sounds. Over time, your focus, concentration and attention span will begin to improve and lengthen.

I want to share some basic techniques with you that really helped me during my first few weeks, but if you're still struggling, you might find it useful to look for a meditation coach or local group practice to get you into the rhythm.

SETTING UP YOUR SPACE

With experience, background noise becomes less of a problem when you meditate, but it can be really beneficial to find a calm, quiet space to begin with. If you have room in your home to set aside an area dedicated to meditation, that's great. It doesn't have to be an entire room, a space in the corner of an existing one will be just fine. That space can serve as a reminder of your intention to practise stillness. You could even set up your meditation space in the backyard or garden during summer. Most importantly it should be somewhere private where you're not going to get disturbed.

You don't need much in your meditation space besides a cosy cushion or blanket – the idea is to keep it simple. But it can be helpful to have a focal point to rest your attention on, something like a little statue or candle.

SIT STILL FOR TWO MINUTES

This might sound ridiculously easy. Your mission to begin with is just to meditate for two minutes every day for a week. If that goes well, increase it by another two minutes and do that for a week. Keep gradually upping your time and you'll be meditating for 10 minutes a day by month two – which is amazing!

Make a commitment to meditate at the same time each day. To keep things simple this might be as soon as you wake up, or just before you go to bed. Keeping your meditation time regular to begin with is all part of forming a positive pattern.

Sit down in your meditation space. It might feel nice to sit cross-legged, or if you struggle with back pain, using a supportive cushion or wall can help. I love to meditate lying down, but I have to force myself not to because I have a tendency to fall asleep! While it's good to relax, dozing off is not the idea.

As you first settle into your meditation session, begin by checking in with how you're feeling. How does your body feel? How does your skin feel? What is your state of mind? Busy? Tired? Stressed? Regard whatever you're bringing to this meditation session as completely okay.

BREATHE

Once you're settled in, turn your attention to your breath. Breathe in deeply through your nose, focus on your breath as it comes in and follow it all the way down into your lungs. In your mind count "one" as you take in the first breath, then "two" as you breathe out. Repeat to the count of ten, then begin again at one.

It is perfectly normal during this practice for all kinds of thoughts to creep in. Remember, this is not about clearing your mind or stopping your thought process. That can sometimes happen, but it's not the "goal" of meditation. When you notice your mind wandering, don't berate yourself. Smile and simply return gently to your breath. Count from one again, starting over. This isn't something to feel frustrated about: it's perfectly normal.

There are lots of brilliant meditation apps and timers available. Guided meditation can offer a fantastic alternative if you're really struggling to begin by yourself or would like to practise for longer with some help.

Please don't let this be a fad you attempt for the next day or two. It's important to really commit yourself to it as stringently as you're committing to diet, exercise and a new skincare regime. Set yourself the target of a month, increasing your daily meditation time by two minutes each week. Meditation isn't always easy, or even peaceful, but it has truly amazing long-term benefits. The best thing is, it's something you can begin to do right away and continue to do for the rest of your life.

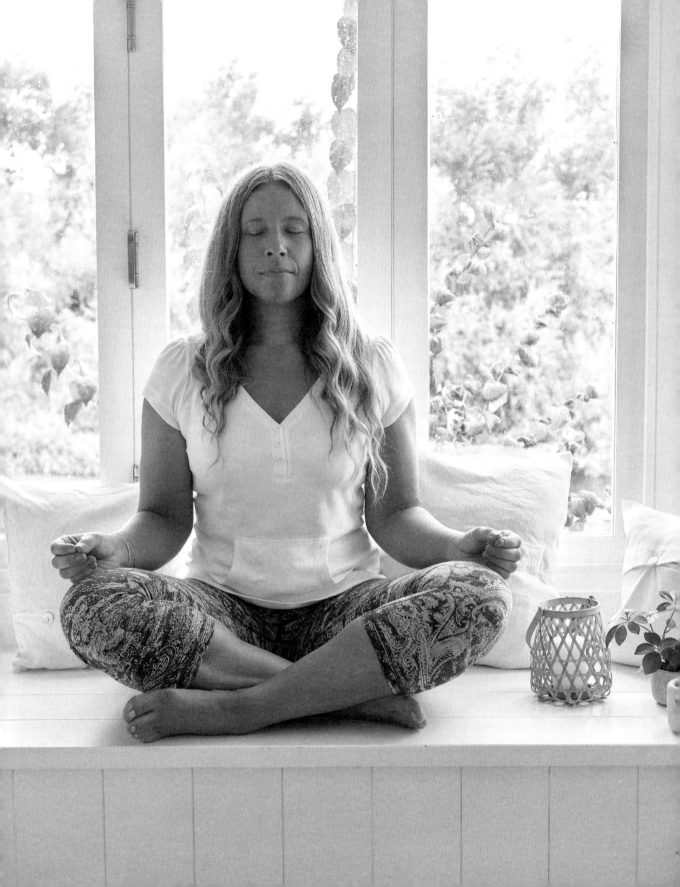

LIVE YOUR
best life

It can sometimes seem as though everyone else in the world has their "best life" formula all figured out. Scroll through social media and you're very often faced with beautiful people boasting perfect skin in itsy-bitsy bikinis striking a pose in the world's most exotic locations. This is not what living your best life is all about. It's more about the everyday little wins that add up to the big stuff. Instagram is not real life and the word "best" is subjective. Strip away the social media filters and look at your true values objectively and with honesty.

For me, the key to living my best life is figuring out the small stuff that makes me smile every day. Getting up before sunrise, exercising often, eating well, exploring new places, simple things like enjoying a relaxing salt bath. It isn't about what everyone else is doing, but more about what matters to me most on an achievable level. Your idea of best might not look like mine – and that's absolutely fine, too.

Take a moment to think about what you really want from your life right now. Once you've got that figured out, it's time to set some intentions. It can sometimes be more helpful to view living our best lives as an ever-evolving process – what's relevant today might not matter to you so much next month or next year. There is always room for improvement – we can continually learn more about ourselves and this self-awareness and growth allows us to progressively become more fulfilled versions of ourselves.

SET YOUR INTENTIONS

Failing to set our intentions is like getting in the car without a clear direction in mind. Don't get me wrong, I love random road trips into the unknown, but that won't serve us well if there's a specific destination we want to get to.

The difference between setting a goal versus setting an intention is that goals are all about accomplishing specific outcomes, whereas an intention is much more focused on achieving a specific mindset or feeling. Setting intentions is more about adjusting the mood and vibe in our brain.

Intentions are also about enjoying the journey. When we pick a goal and resolutely focus on achieving it, we can sometimes make ourselves miserable along the way. If our goal is clear skin, for example, and we see new spots arising while we're detoxing, we might immediately think we've failed. If, however, our intention is to learn to be calm, comfortable and healthy in our own skin, we are much more likely to enjoy the different stages of that journey. Above all, intention setting should be enjoyable and sustainable.

WORDS OF ALIGNMENT

Begin by writing a list of words that resonate with how you'd like to feel. This can really help to keep you on track when you're feeling lost or stuck. Remember, your intentions do not have to be the same as mine, your partner's or anybody else's and they're not set in stone. Intentions can change and evolve over time. Having a list to draw from can be a brilliant starting point to simplify the process.

VISUALIZE THE PROCESS

We're so used to enjoying the experience of a feeling as a result of something we've achieved, that we forget it's entirely possible to manifest the feeling first and accomplish great things as a result. Why should we have to wait to feel how we want? Switch things around. Think about how you would feel with clear skin. Confident? Happy? Free? Now focus on manifesting those feelings first.

WRITE DOWN YOUR INTENTIONS

The most effective way to set, maintain and track our intentions can be to write them down and say them out loud. Use a journal to list your wishes and keep up to date with progress or obstacles.

This year I shall:
» Embrace …
» Love …
» Share …
» Focus more on …
» Take extra time to …
» Learn about …
» Release my fear of …

QUESTIONS TO CONSIDER

» What does happiness look like to you?
» Is there one big goal you have for this year?
» In what ways would you like to improve your health?
» Are there new skills that you'd like to learn?
» What do you consider yourself to be good at?
» What new routines would you like to incorporate into your daily life over the coming months?
» What big changes would you make if fear wasn't holding you back?

The goal of exploring intentions is not to create more demands or pressure in your life. Don't beat yourself up if you're struggling to complete the exercise. I don't want this to add more stress to your journey. The purpose is more to shed light and this might be an ongoing process. You can always come back to it when you feel ready. Trust the process, practise gratitude each day (see page 139) and reach for good-feeling thoughts.

There is always room for improvement – we can continually learn more about ourselves

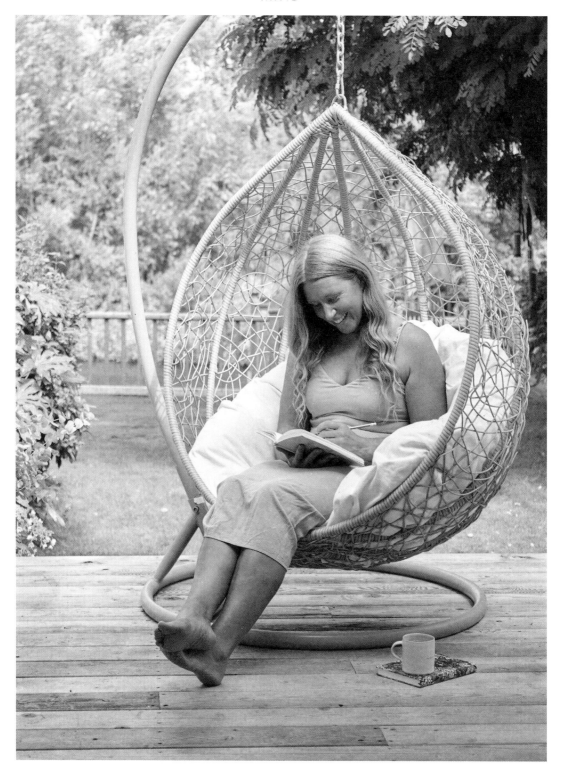

GRATITUDE

Practising gratitude can have a truly significant impact on our wellbeing. Taking time to notice and reflect upon the things we are most thankful for helps us experience more positive emotions, feel alive, sleep better, express more compassion and kindness, and as a result, build a strong gut microbiome and healthy immune system.

There are lots of ways in which we can practise gratitude. Being more mindful by reminding ourselves of the good things in our lives is a brilliant first step. Talking to ourselves in a positive way in the mirror each morning is another. Writing down our thoughts takes gratitude one step further. Gratitude journalling works because it slowly changes the way we perceive situations by adjusting our focus. Rather than thinking of our skin as this awful thing that brings us misery, work on changing your perspective to think about it like Danielle does (see page 128), as something that protects you, covers your bones and muscles, something that acts as an early warning system – a very visible barometer of health. I know it's difficult to think positively about something that has brought you a great deal of misery, but this all important change in mindset can make a huge difference.

GRATITUDE JOURNAL

Keeping a gratitude journal is a beautifully simple way to record all the things for which we're grateful. It can travel with us anywhere, making it easy to note our gratitude daily. Everyone's journal will be different. Finding time to write in it can be difficult at first. Try to associate it with an existing habit – when you drink your Liver Cleanse Tea (see page 122)

for example, or as part of your bedtime routine before you doze off at night. Just pick your time and stick to it.

Here are some examples of things you might like to journal about:

» Think about something unique about you for which you're grateful.
» What made you laugh out loud this week?
» Name somebody who did something kind for you. What did they do?
» If you could choose to keep only three things you own, what would you choose and why?
» Scroll back through your photos and write about a memory for which you're grateful.
» List five things that made you happy this week.
» Think about something kind you've done for somebody else.
» Write about a friend for whom you are truly grateful.
» Reflect on a mistake or something that went wrong and how you dealt with it positively.
» What do you love about your surroundings?
» What was the highlight of your week?
» What natural talent or skill do you have for which you're grateful?

DISCONNECT
& reconnect

In today's tech-heavy world, it can quickly become habit to begin and end the day staring at your phone, without really noticing the environment around you. Stepping away from technology and into nature has been proven to recharge and restore our sense of health and wellbeing.

I'm not a big fan of cycling at the gym or running on the treadmill, but when it comes to getting on my bike outdoors or running in the hills, I absolutely love it. It's about boosting my mental wellbeing as well as my physical wellbeing. Scientific research reveals that spending time in nature, breathing in fresh air and surrounding ourselves with flora and fauna can significantly reduce levels of stress and anxiety. The action of deeply breathing fresh oxygen can positively impact the levels of serotonin produced in our brain and, as we know, serotonin is key to boosting feelings of happiness and relaxation. I love to ensure my skin is getting gradual, gentle doses of vitamin D. Is there a biking trail you can go on? A park you can run through? A beach you can walk along? Spending time in nature and embracing the benefits can bring us great happiness and joy. How will you get offline and get outside to embrace time in nature this week?

LEARNING FOR LIFE

Learning enables us to grow. We learn new things on a daily basis, as our interactions, experiences and relationships continually teach us. We can also choose to actively add to our education through listening to podcasts, attending events, watching movies, reading books and connecting with people on a similar path. Opening ourselves up to new experiences when we're on a holistic quest to health and wellbeing can really help us focus on positive new hobbies, creating a distraction from perhaps less conducive old ones. Many of my weekend social events used to involve alcohol! Stepping away from Saturday afternoon drinking sessions and prioritizing simple new experiences, such as swimming in open water or camping at a weekend food festival, most certainly helped me realize what was truly important in my life and that in turn helped me to become more mindful. When we're working to make great changes to our health and skin, educating and empowering ourselves can give us back a sense of control. This helps us to fulfil our potential and set goals that are important to us to create a life we love.

Write down a list of inspirational movies and books you'd like to watch and read. Take a look online for local festivals, groups or wellbeing events that can give you the opportunity to learn and connect with like-minded people.

MOVIES:

BOOKS:

EVENTS:

BEGIN YOUR DAY BETTER

How many mornings recently have you woken up late, reached for your phone, scrolled absent-mindedly through social media, reluctantly rolled out of bed, skipped breakfast and rushed to work? Whether you're a night owl or a morning person, embracing an inspiring and productive morning routine will set you up for a productive and inspiring day.

It might feel really difficult at first, getting up an hour earlier to make time for a healthy start, but consistent morning rituals will eventually become second nature. Exercising first thing, making time for meditation, writing in your journal, enjoying a nutritious breakfast and taking a moment to enjoy a cup of skin purifying tea are lovely ways to relax, reflect and centre your mind, helping you to make the most of the day ahead.

Just as a set bedtime routine can help to get us into a regular pattern of sleeping well, an established morning routine can be equally beneficial, to get us used to a consistent pattern of beginning the day well. Write down your new planned morning routine.

MORNING ROUTINE:

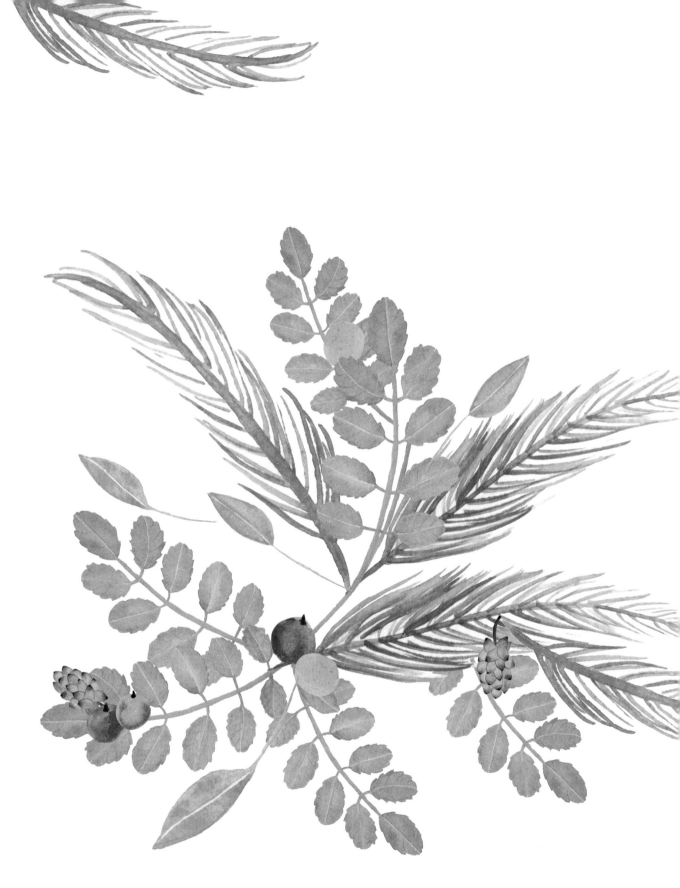

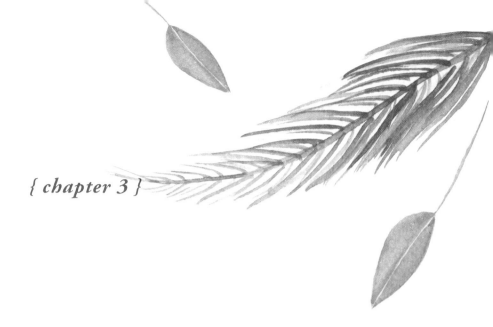

exercise

It might seem a bit confusing at first, making the connection between exercise and our skin. Why would a workout make the slightest bit of difference to your skin condition? When we think of exercise we usually associate it with getting fit, losing weight or gaining muscle, but exercise is also vital for skin health.

When we exercise, blood flows to the surface of our skin. I recall my skin looking bright red and angry after jogging. It felt more painful than ever and that always put me off making exercise a regular thing. Rosacea might redden, psoriasis and eczema patches can look inflamed, but this is temporary and is actually a positive. The long-term benefits of exercise far outweigh the short-term flare. By increasing blood flow, exercise helps nourish skin cells. In addition to providing oxygen, blood flow also helps carry away waste products, including free radicals, from working cells. Sweat is great for clearing skin! It purges the body of toxins that can clog pores and lead to acne. Exercise allows sweat glands to up their function and get rid of those toxins. Your cells also start producing more of their natural oils, helping skin look healthy and naturally hydrated.

EXERCISE *&* GUT

I keep coming back to gut wellbeing because I believe it's absolutely integral to the health of our skin. Scientists investigating the microbiome are learning more and more each year. Although it's a relatively new area of research, studies are continually emerging exploring the correlation between exercise and the trillions of bacteria living in our digestive tract. Without getting too scientific, short-chain fatty acids have been shown to increase during cardio exercise. This in turn can strengthen the gut. A 30-minute session of moderate exercise can stimulate the immune system, producing an anti-inflammatory response. Just this half hour of moderate exercise (including fast walking) is sufficient to achieve results.

EXERCISE & THE LYMPHATIC SYSTEM

You might have heard about the body's lymphatic system, but have absolutely no idea what it actually does. In comparison to our digestive system or our nervous system, it's much less referenced or talked about, but when it comes to fighting chronic skin disease, its functioning is vital. The lymph consists of vessels and tissues, which are similar to the veins and capillaries we see in our circulatory system. But instead of pumping blood around the body, our lymphatic system is tasked with carrying away and filtering waste. Our spleen, lymph nodes, tonsils and lymphatic tissues in the bowel are all connected to this intricate system.

Scientists are increasingly exploring the link between strep throat infections, inflammatory bowel disease and psoriasis. You might notice yourself a correlation between recurring sore throats, tonsillitis or Crohn's Disease and ulcerative colitis contributing to your skin flares – in this instance, looking after your lymph is even more vital. A weakened lymphatic system can compromise our immunity, meaning we're more susceptible to getting run-down and sick, so it's vital for us to eat well and move well in order to help it do its job properly.

Poor lymph circulation can lead to inflammation and chronic skin disease. A combination of a sedentary lifestyle, unhealthy diet, and a toxic environment all contribute to this backup. Constant fatigue, chronic skin problems, recurrent sore throats, worsened allergies, itching and sinus infections might indicate a stagnant lymphatic system. Rapid improvements in the quality of our cells and blood occur once

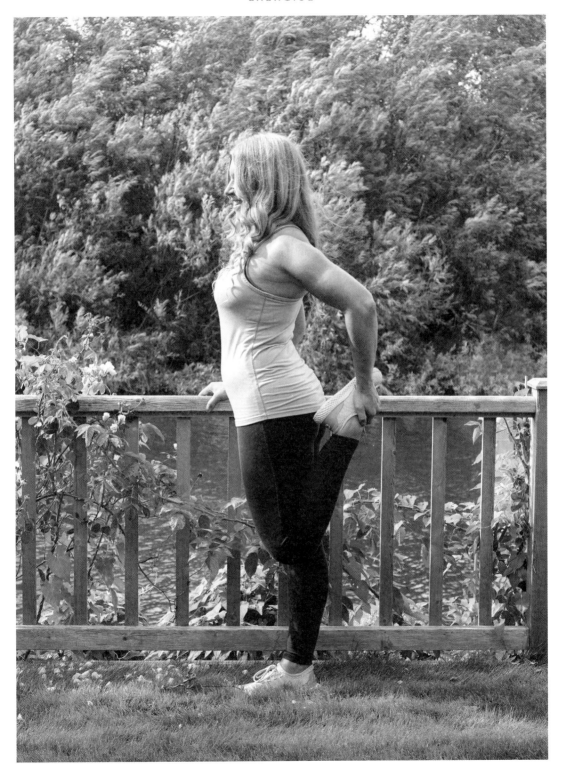

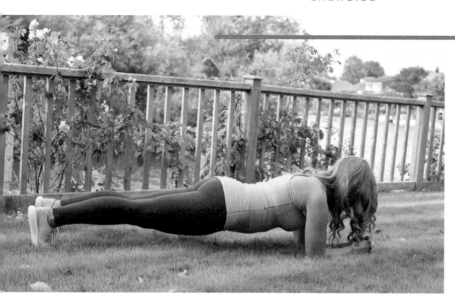

The initial mission is to get your body moving

simple lifestyle changes are made, so that the lymphatic system is reactivated to work efficiently again.

Breathing deeply, proper hydration and muscle activity in the body are all key factors for healthy lymphatic function. If you think about it, when we participate in cardiovascular exercise such as running or cycling, we typically provide all three. If these activities feel a bit too much for you, don't worry – gentle yoga stretches can offer a great alternative. Holding stretches combined with conscious deep breathing can help direct lymph through the channels of the chest.

GETTING STARTED

Whether you're incorporating regular exercise into your routine for the first time, or easing back into exercise after a break, start small. Commit to just fifteen minutes of walking, cycling or stretching for three days this week. This will help create the good habits you want to have in place.

The reality of embarking on any journey, whether it's business, relationships, diet, or fitness, is you're going to make mistakes and stumble along the way. There will naturally be

times when the roller coaster of life gets crazy and you may feel momentarily derailed. The difference between failing and succeeding, as with so many things in life, is that you have the option to pick yourself up from the fall and keep going, or use it as an easy excuse to quit. Just like you would if you were faced with an issue at work, identify the problem and take action to make sure it doesn't throw you off course next time.

ADVANCE PLANNING

If you're picking mornings as your time to train, pack up your gym bag or prepare anything else you need, like setting out your water bottle and trainers the night before. If you'd rather work out in the afternoon and your lifestyle allows it, consider wearing your workout clothes during that day when you're running errands or taking the kids to school. Having everything ready to go will make it so much easier to get yourself to work out. Advance planning can eliminate decisions about your workout, your clothes, or what you're eating that day and it will put you in the mindset that this workout will happen.

WHAT TO WEAR

Skin conditions can make exercise very painful. If you're really struggling with sore skin, wearing soft, comfortable clothing can help. While for most people fashion and cost are the only considerations when buying new clothes, for many of us with chronic skin conditions, shopping is more stressful. Look for soft cotton and seam-free clothes. Don't worry about wearing tight-fitting lycra, go with what's comfortable for you – if that's an old baggy t-shirt and soft jogging bottoms, who cares?

HOW SHOULD I EXERCISE?

Whether you run, dance, swim, bike, box or lift … it really doesn't matter. The initial mission is to get your body moving. If that's something you haven't done in quite a while, you might want to start off with something as gentle as a walk in nature, or a beginner's yoga class.

The type of exercise you want to do depends very much on what you enjoy. That is the most important consideration – exercise has got to be fun! Of course, there are going to be times when we'd prefer crashing on the sofa with a movie and takeaway but if you choose something you have some level of interest in, that's a much stronger starting point.

I'm constantly changing what I do to keep things interesting. Last year it was boxing, the year before that I was out on my paddleboard all the time. This year it's triathlons and endurance training outdoors. I can't say what I'll be doing next year because if I begin to feel as though it's a constant bind to go out and exercise, that's when I know I need a change.

SET GOALS

Setting goals really helps you to stay motivated and on track. I like to challenge myself to compete. I am by no means the fastest, but I love the atmosphere of a race day. The people who take part in these events and the marshals are so lovely, I massively look forward to them. Bear in mind, my starting point was the local 5km park run – and I spent my first few attempts walking most of that! The challenge you set yourself does not have to be huge, but having a goal in mind gives you a purpose and that's what inspires you on those mornings when you'd rather have an extra hour in bed.

ROPE IN FRIENDS AND FAMILY

I'm very fortunate, as my running buddy James lives literally next door. I'll go out and exercise on my own too, but having a friend you can train with is massive for accountability and motivation. There are plenty of days when I'll message to say "Come on, let's get out there!" and similarly times when I've felt lazy but a message to say "Let's go!" has been the difference between bothering with a 5km run and making excuses to stay in bed.

Exercise does not have to be a compromise between family time and training: I'll often take my little godson, Jack, out on his bike or for a trek through the forest at weekends. We'll go and do a 10km circuit around the lake. Jack loves the chance to have a muddy adventure, while I remind myself that exercise really needn't feel like exercise at all. In summer we'll pick hedgerow berries, in autumn we'll go out searching for conkers, and before you know it we've walked 10,000 steps and it hasn't even begun to feel like exercise! Get the kids involved, ask your partner to join you on a hilly hike; there are so many brilliant family events at weekends.

STAYING ACCOUNTABLE

Most of us set out on our health and wellbeing journey eager and full of enthusiasm. We can't wait to get started and begin making changes right away. Unfortunately, this new-found motivation can tend to dwindle. Before long we start to flake and miss the odd session here and there. We have a tough day at work and would rather head straight home and chill out than go for a run. Or hit that snooze button instead of getting up and putting on our trainers at 6am. These "odd" missed sessions soon add up and before we know it, we haven't worked out for a fortnight.

Accountability is something we all need at times. Think back to school. What motivated you to finish your homework? Was it a love of learning? Knowing how valuable this skill was going to be in the future? I expect it was more likely the threat of getting detention if you failed to hand it in on time!

Accountability is exactly what it sounds like, someone keeping you accountable for what you're doing. That someone might be a coach, it might be a friend, a stranger or family member, or it might be you. Staying accountable to ourselves requires a serious amount of commitment. When the only person holding you accountable to your workouts is yourself, it becomes too easy to skip your session. There have been numerous studies conducted into accountability over the years, all of which demonstrate how being accountable to someone else far improves your chances of success. It's so easy to fall off the wagon and

willpower will only go so far. However, if you add somebody else into the equation to keep you accountable, you are much more likely to succeed.

Accountability can be lots of different things; sharing progress on social media, keeping a wellness journal or signing up with a coach or app – all of which can keep you on track and remind you to keep going!

DO SOMETHING DIFFERENT

When you think about exercise, your immediate thought might be "I hate the gym!". Exercise does not have to involve a gym, a running track or a pool. Why not look for something different? An open water swimming group, salsa classes, white-water rafting! Anything to get out there and get your body moving. I love to combine exercise with time in nature. It resets my mood and helps my mental wellbeing as much as my physical health.

It might be that you're often pushed for time in your busy schedule. In that case, there are plenty of simple ways to incorporate movement into your regular daily routine. Walking the kids to school, cycling to work, taking the stairs; simple every day changes that will get the lymphatic system moving.

REMEMBER WHY YOU STARTED
When it comes to achieving your goals ... don't just set them and forget them. Remind yourself regularly why your goal is important to you. Subtle sticky note reminders can help you stay focused. It could be a memo on your laptop with the goal itself written on it or an inspirational quote scribbled down as encouragement. Or you could make the screen saver on your phone a picture of that sleeveless outfit you dream of wearing or the beach you want to feel comfortable relaxing on with your family. Keep these reminders front and centre so you see them when you lack incentive or feel ready to quit.

KATE'S STORY

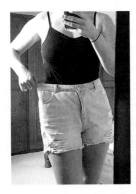

"I've never had perfect skin and always envied anyone that did. Whenever I've been ill, the first place it shows up is my skin. I have really sensitive skin and it's got worse as I've grown older.

Until this year I hadn't even heard of guttate psoriasis, so when I got a strep throat infection and broke out in a rash, I couldn't figure out what it was. When the doctor confirmed my diagnosis, I was worried. They offered me a cream, but I was concerned that it might make things worse.

I'd already promised myself, as I did every New Year, that I would make changes to my health and diet. I began researching anti-inflammatory diets and that's where I came across Hanna's book. I'm such a foodie, so I was pleasantly surprised to realise just how tasty this lifestyle looked. My partner and I now make everything from scratch. We've even started growing our own organic vegetables!

What I found really helpful when I started making these changes was learning about why they were so beneficial for me. It helped me to feel educated and empowered, to know how this was going to help change my health and skin.

Now I'm actually grateful for that flare-up in January, because it prompted a massive positive lifestyle change. I've also lost two stone. I love my new lifestyle and I'm in no hurry to slip back into old habits."

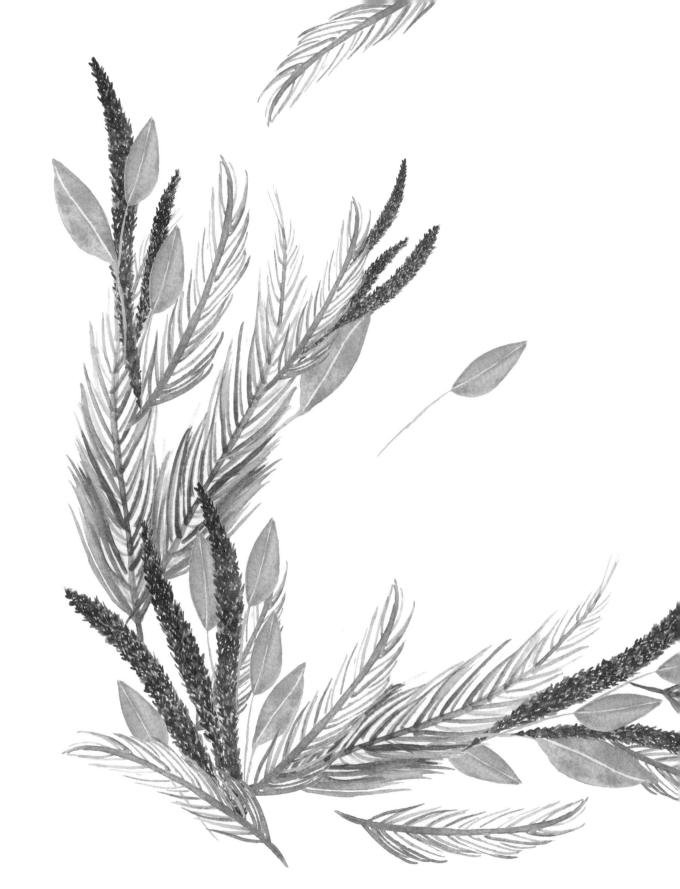

sleep

When it comes to getting a good night's sleep, its impact on our gut bacteria, and in turn our skin, is increasingly being seen as a two-way street. Our gut microbiome seems to play a role in how well we sleep, but sleep and circadian rhythms also appear to affect the health and diversity of the important bacterial world that lives in our gut.

Dealing with a skin condition can massively impact your sleep. If skin feels tight, sore or itchy, it can prevent you from sleeping or wake you up in the middle of the night. Not enough, inconsistent or poor-quality sleep are all linked to an increased risk of chronic health conditions. A good night's sleep, on the other hand, can make you feel good, reduce stress levels and promote positive health changes.

Melatonin, a sleep hormone primarily produced by the pineal gland, is responsible for managing the body's circadian rhythm. In the gut, a substance called tryptophan can be converted to melatonin to help regulate the sleep–wake cycle. However, this requires the gut to function properly. A poorly functioning or compromised gut could well be responsible for your insomnia.

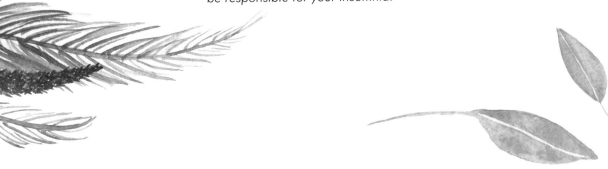

BEDTIME *routine*

Do you have a bedtime routine? You might remember how strict your bedtime routine was as a child. You'd go upstairs at a set time each evening, brush your teeth, put on your pyjamas, have a story read to you (if you were lucky!) and drift off peacefully. That routine stayed consistent, regardless of the time of year.

As adults, our evening routine seems to go completely out of the window at times. Even if you have a sort-of set bedtime each night, I'm betting it invariably changes throughout the week. Social events, work deadlines, evenings out … there are lots of things that disrupt our best-laid plans.

If you struggle to doze off, it's extra important to stick to the same sleep schedule every night, so your body can find its natural rhythm and settle into a regular sleep–wake cycle.

As well as throwing your body out of sync, an irregular sleep schedule can impact the quality of sleep you're getting, meaning you never enter the stages of deep sleep your brain and body need to restore themselves.

Whether you're a night owl or an early bird is largely irrelevant; the key is consistency. Set a time you'd like to go to sleep and make this a priority. If that time is 9pm, ensure you're in bed, lights out, ready to drift off to sleep by 9pm every night.

WRITE OUT YOUR NEW BEDTIME ROUTINE

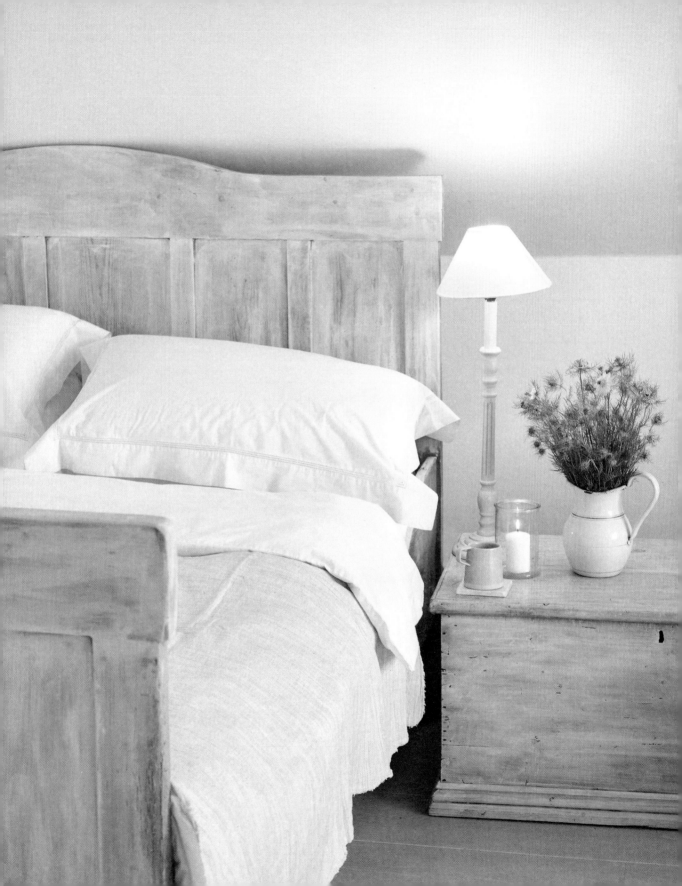

TECH

What is the very last thing you do before going to sleep? It might be telling your partner you love them, it could be reading a book, but more often than not it involves staring at a screen. In an ideal world, screens would be banned from the bedroom, but these days our phones are our everything. What if somebody needs to reach us in an emergency? What would we do without three alarms and a snooze function? We always have an excuse that pretty much keeps our phone surgically attached to our hand. If you're not quite ready for a full digital detox just yet, at least ensure that you've set your smartphone to switch to night mode an hour before you're due to sleep. This filters the screen to eliminate blue light that interferes with our circadian rhythm. Try to limit screen time before you sleep and do something more productive when you wake up (like a two-minute meditation) before you begin scrolling social media and checking emails. It's a difficult habit to get out of, but can make a huge difference to your morning and night-time routines.

ENVIRONMENT

Creating an environment conducive to a good night's sleep might seem logical, and even a little simplistic, but it really can be the difference between struggling to drift off and snoozing soundly. Sleeping in a chaotic, cluttered bedroom reinforces stress and turmoil. Ensure your bedroom is a quiet, clean, enjoyable space. Lights, noise and temperature can all play a role, too.

A comfortable mattress goes without saying. We've all slept in that hotel room, which was lovely … if only the mattress had been firmer / softer / squishier (delete as applicable). Duvets, sheets and pillows also matter, especially when it comes to our skin. Choosing anti-allergy bedding and breathable cotton bed sheets can really make a difference to our levels of cosiness.

ESSENTIAL OILS

Strong scents can have a significant impact on how we feel. When we smell something, a signal goes straight to our limbic system and amygdala (the parts of our brain responsible for our memory or mood). Choosing scents that promote relaxation can help get our bodies into a restful state ready for sleep. There are a number of ways in which you can use essential oils to help you get a better night's sleep. Simply adding a few drops on to your pillow can be very effective. You might like to use them in a warm bath an hour or so before bed, or combine them into a scented pillow spray.

Lavender calms the nervous system by lowering blood pressure, heart rate and skin temperature, helping to put your body in a state conducive to sleep.

Valerian root can be used as a herbal tea or essential oil. It contains valerenic acid, which produces the natural sedative effects for which the root is known.

Ensure your bedroom is a quiet, clean, enjoyable space

Chamomile tea is well renowned for its calming properties. Chamomile oil works in exactly the same way, lowering stress and anxiety. It has even been said to reduce nightmares!

Jasmine is such a lovely, floral fragrance. Studies show it's linked to reduced anxiety levels and can improve sleep quality as a result.

Geranium is considered to have a gently relaxing effect on the mood and works as a natural antidepressant.

SLEEPY TEA

These are my absolute favourite herbs to use in a bedtime tea blend, not just in the evening but also as a lovely, calming cuppa whenever life gets hectic or stressful. Each herb has specific properties conducive to restful sleep, a healthy gut and, in turn, clear skin.

Try concocting your own sleepy blends using the herbs below.

Chamomile flower has been used as a natural remedy to reduce inflammation, decrease anxiety and treat insomnia.

Valerian root has a long history of usefulness as a natural sleep aid and anti-anxiety remedy.

Passionflower appears to boost the level of gamma-aminobutyric acid (GABA) in your brain. This compound lowers brain activity, which may help you relax and sleep.

Lime flower is a traditional remedy for nightmares and bad dreams. Its calming effect on the nervous system also makes it effective in treating a nervous digestion.

Rose tea (blossoms or petals) has a natural sedative property that makes helps reduce inflammation, ease stress and regulate hormones related to circadian rhythm and sleep pattern.

Lavender flower has a wonderful ability to induce calm.

Lemon balm reduces stress and anxiety.

MAGNESIUM

Magnesium is a mineral involved in hundreds of processes in the human body, and is important for brain function and heart health. In addition, magnesium may help quiet the mind and body, making it easier to fall asleep. Studies show that magnesium's relaxing effect may be partly due to its ability to regulate the production of melatonin, a hormone that guides your body's sleep–wake cycle. Studies report that insufficient levels of magnesium in your body may be linked to troubled sleep and insomnia. On the other hand, increasing your magnesium intake by taking supplements may help you optimize the quality and quantity of your sleep.

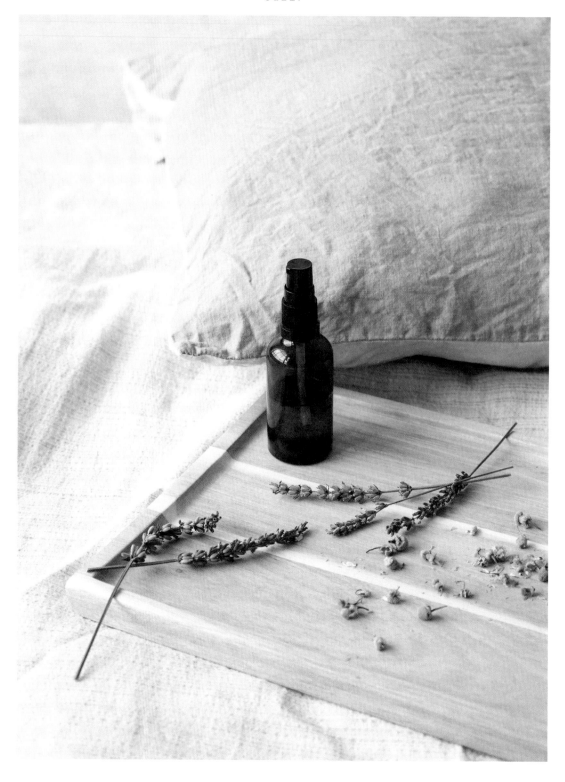

SOOTHING
pillow spray

Aromatherapy oils are a wonderful sensory tool to help encourage a peaceful night's sleep. Spraying a few drops of this pillow spray close to your head, as part of a bedtime routine, can help you to fall asleep faster and wake up feeling refreshed.

Makes 60ml (2fl oz)

½ **teaspoon witch hazel**
4 **drops chamomile essential oil**
12 **drops lavender essential oil**
8 **drops jasmine essential oil**
50ml (1¾fl oz) **distilled water**

Put the witch hazel and essential oils into a 60ml (2fl oz) sterilized glass spray bottle and swirl to combine. Add the water and close the spray bottle. Shake well to combine.

To use the spray, lightly mist a pillow a few minutes before bedtime. Ensure you shake the bottle well before each use.

I keep my pillow spray in my bedside drawer out of direct sunlight for up to 3 months.

Scents that promote relaxation get our bodies ready for sleep

skincare

Since my protocol and everything I coach centres around what we're putting into our bodies, why should it matter what we're applying on to the surface of our skin? Trust me, it matters. Don't let your clean living be ruined by toxins absorbed externally.

Think about a nicotine patch. Its purpose is to feed nicotine directly into the bloodstream through the skin. If nicotine can enter the body in such a concentrated form, then rest assured that chemicals massaged routinely and deeply into the skin most certainly can too.

INCI names (International Nomenclature Cosmetic Ingredient – those funny, Latin-looking words you see listed in the ingredients on skincare products) can make labels difficult to understand. There are many chemical-sounding ingredients that show up on our skincare labels that might sound dangerous or strange. However, the old adage of "it's not safe if you can't pronounce it" is not a great way to vet things. The truth is, everything is made up of chemicals: water, soil, plants, even us! So, instead of saying "avoid chemicals", what we actually mean is "avoid harsh or harmful chemicals".

There is a reason natural skincare is costlier and it isn't just because the manufacturers believe the words "natural" or "organic" warrant an excessive price hike! Natural skincare is pricey to manufacture. Without the inclusion of cheap preservatives, surfactants and foaming agents, these products are simply more expensive to produce. Cheap products are cheap because they use cheap ingredients, and these ingredients are not always kind to our skin. Invest in yourself, your health and your skin by not skimping on skincare.

THE BAD

Let's take, for example, one of the most commonly used ingredients I see in mainstream skincare, including in creams labelled as "suitable for eczema and sensitive skin". You might notice it in the lotion you're using right now, labelled as "mineral oil", "paraffin" or "paraffinum liquidum"… It's essentially the same thing: petrol. Besides the obvious conclusion that highly refined petrol is not going to benefit anybody in the long run, this also makes many of our most commonly used skincare products highly flammable. If clothing, bandages or dressings soaked in cream come into contact with an open flame or heat source, it can easily ignite. Between 2010 and 2017, 37 deaths in the UK have been attributed to this exact same scenario. Devastating for something that can be easily avoided.

Besides this horrible statistic, paraffin can be hugely problematic for those of us with sensitive skin. It's in pretty much every emollient recommended or prescribed for dry skin, eczema or psoriasis, and it's in most high street hand creams and moisturizers too. It's used because it's cheap – being a byproduct of the oil industry.

The reason it is found in so many products is that it is the cheapest way to resolve the immediate problem of dryness, but what about the long-term problems that might ensue?

Paraffin provides a thin, oily, protective layer on the skin, so that when the skin's own barrier is weak, broken or faulty, it can be protected against allergens and irritants, while locking moisture into the skin where it's needed.

By itself, paraffin is greasy, unpleasant smelling and not very nice to use, so manufacturers often add preservatives and strong fragrance-masking chemicals to paraffin to make it useable – these can also cause irritation to sensitive skin. Regardless of these additives, paraffin can cause irritation and inflammation all by itself. It forms an occlusive (waterproof) barrier over the skin, which means it can clog pores and cause breakouts in oily or acne-prone skin. That occlusive barrier doesn't allow our skin to breathe, so it can't shed waste products as it would naturally. Essentially, these creams lock in dirt as well as moisture, which increases the risk of bacterial and fungal infection.

Besides these very obvious considerations, there are also concerns that using an occlusive barrier over a long period of time reduces our skin's ability to function normally and to regenerate itself.

PARABENS

Parabens were first introduced into cosmetics in the 1950s. They're an inexpensive and common type of preservative designed to kill bacteria and microorganisms in our skincare products. When we're dipping dirty fingertips into our face cream each morning, preservatives are essential to stop that dirt growing into a fungus. Sound amazing, don't they? That is until you realize they are endocrine disruptors that can confuse hormone function by mimicking oestrogen.

Endocrine disruptors are chemicals that may interfere with the body's hormone system and produce adverse developmental, reproductive, neurological, and immune effects in both humans and wildlife. In the past decade, scientists have found that the number of environmental contaminants with oestrogen-like properties is much greater than they had imagined. Parabens are synthetic oestrogens, meaning that they behave like oestrogen in the body, in turn disrupting our own natural hormone system.

The US Environmental Protection Agency (EPA) has even linked methyl-parabens, in particular, to metabolic, developmental, hormonal, and neurological disorders, as well as various cancers.

The good news is that parabens can be found clearly labelled in the product's ingredient list. Here's what to look for (and avoid):

- Methylparaben
- Butylparaben
- Propylparaben
- Ethylparaben
- Isobutylparaben
- Benzylparaben

Essential oil extracts and certain herbs can act as a natural preservative. They don't possess the toxicity of their paraben counterparts but they remain effective. That said, oils can break down much more quickly, which is why some natural skincare manufacturers advise storing your lotion in the refrigerator. Natural preservatives usually need to be used in larger concentrations, which can also make the product more expensive.

SLS

SLS, or Sodium Lauryl Sulphate to give it its full name, is another ingredient that's been given a bad rap of late – and with good reason. This is the stuff that makes your bath foam go foamy, and helps your shampoo to lather. Prolonged use has been shown to increase skin sensitivity – including irritation, dryness and itching. If you struggle with scalp psoriasis or dermatitis, you don't need me to tell you that massaging this into an already irritated and inflamed scalp is not going to be conducive to healing.

Paraffin, parabens and SLS are just small examples of the worst offenders when it comes to problematic ingredients in our cosmetics. I could go on but let's instead focus on the good stuff we should be applying to our skin and move on to some easy homemade recipes, which will make applying these beneficial ingredients simple.

THE GOOD

It can feel very disappointing when you learn about the cheap ingredients that are so often used in the manufacture of mainstream skincare products. Even those supposedly designed for very sensitive skin often contain something we should probably avoid in the long run.

I remember feeling that disappointment when I realized that most of the products I'd been applying daily – including what I thought was a natural scar minimizing oil – contained petrol in some form or another. The ingredients list on the back of the skincare I'd been slathering on for years made for very depressing reading.

The real learning curve came when I made the decision to develop my own skincare range, based on everything I'd learned over the years. I was struggling to find natural, affordable products in the shops suitable for my problem skin. Anything I did come across looked so clinical and bland. Scalp treatments stank of coal tar and nothing ticked all the boxes. I wanted to incorporate all those amazing natural botanicals that had massively helped me over the years. I spent a long time developing a declarable allergen-free fragrance that works as a generic male or female scent – something natural and herbal without smelling overpowering or sickly sweet. Most of all, I dreamt of beautiful products, full of wonderful ingredients, that I could display proudly in my bathroom, because I'd spent so many years hiding the stuff I was using in bedroom drawers to avoid awkward questions from friends about my skin.

You can find out more about my range at www.hannasillitoe.com.

CARRIER OILS

Essential oils can be fantastic when it comes to caring for our skin, but they are volatile, meaning they evaporate quickly, leaving behind a concentrated potent aroma. This often makes them too strong to apply directly to our skin. Carrier oils are the perfect companion for essential oils. They "carry" all the medicinal properties of essential oils through the skin. Using a carrier when making your oil blend gives you full control of concentration levels. Carrier oils have their own therapeutic properties based on the essential fatty acids and natural nutrients they contain.

COCONUT

This is my favourite antioxidant, antifungal, anti-inflammatory and antibacterial body oil. I love how it nourishes my hair, nails and skin. Its almost 50 per cent content of lauric acid means that coconut oil has a long shelf life.

OLIVE OIL

Olive oil is such an easy go-to. You can use it for almost any skin or hair type and it doesn't clog pores or leave skin feeling too greasy. It's an excellent scalp treatment for flaky skin, frizzy hair and dry follicles.

JOJOBA OIL

Jojoba is favoured as the carrier oil that most closely mimics the natural oil secretions of human skin. This makes it an excellent moisturizer for the face and neck that can sometimes feel too greasy with other oils.

ALMOND OIL

Almond oil's high vitamin E content makes it the best choice for nourishing very dry skin, regenerating new skin cells and locking in moisture. I add it to my Dead Sea salt baths to leave skin feeling nourished and hydrated.

ARGAN OIL

Brilliant for healing inflammation and sun damage, argan oil can help reduce the appearance of stretch marks and scars. It's an excellent choice for use on the face and also for nails and nail cuticles.

AVOCADO OIL

Anti-inflammatory and packed with vitamins A, D and E, this is ideal for skin conditions such as psoriasis, dermatitis and eczema.

GRAPESEED OIL

Non-greasy grapeseed oil has antiseptic properties and is a mild astringent, making it a good carrier oil for acne-prone or oily skin.

APRICOT KERNEL OIL

The non-greasy properties of apricot oil make it a good carrier oil to use for oily facial skin, as well as dry, irritated or sensitive skin.

CASTOR OIL

Castor oil can enhance immunity through improving the lymphatic system, which in turn helps the body to detoxify, positively impacting circulation and supporting the digestive tract.

BLACK SEED OIL

Black seed oil contains powerful antioxidants and antibacterial compounds that help strengthen follicles and encourage hair growth. Its anti-inflammatory properties can work to alleviate dandruff and promote a healthy scalp.

HEMP SEED OIL

A brilliant, non-greasy, anti-inflammatory oil that has valuable antioxidant properties, which help with skin cell regeneration and preventing premature ageing. Hemp seed oil is also a natural analgesic (pain-reliever).

HYDRATING
body cream

Makes 135g (4¾oz)

125g (4½oz) shea butter
2 tablespoons jojoba oil

OPTIONAL
10 drops lavender essential oil
5 drops rosemary essential oil
3 drops carrot seed essential oil
3 drops tea tree essential oil

Boil a pan of water and reduce to a simmer. Place a glass bowl on top and melt the shea butter in the bowl over the simmering water. Add the jojoba oil and turn off the heat.

Pour into a clean bowl. Place in the refrigerator or freezer for 15 minutes to cool and return to a solid form.

Once opaque and slightly firm, remove the bowl from the refrigerator or freezer and add the essential oils, if using. Using an electric whisk, whip up the mixture. This takes just a few seconds. Scoop into a wide 150ml (5fl oz) sterilized jar and store in the refrigerator for up to 1 month. Apply to the face and body as desired.

HANDWASH

Makes 375ml (12½fl oz)

350ml (12fl oz) distilled or boiled water (tap water is okay if it will be used within a few weeks)
2 tablespoons liquid Castile soap
½ teaspoon liquid carrier oil (try olive, almond or jojoba)
6 drops essential oils of choice, for scent (optional)

Fill a 375ml (12½fl oz) sterilized soap dispenser to about 2.5cm (1 inch) from the top with the water, leaving room for the pump and the soap to be added.

Add at least 2 tablespoons of liquid Castile soap to the water mixture (don't start with the soap and add water or you will get bubbles). Add the liquid carrier oil and any essential oils, if you are using them.

Close and lightly swoosh around to mix. Use as you would any regular hand soap. Use within 1 month.

GENTLE
chamomile cleanser

Makes about 300ml (10fl oz)

> 1 chamomile tea bag (for its anti-inflammatory properties)
> 250ml (8½fl oz) liquid Castile soap
> 2 tablespoons grapeseed oil
> 10 drops chamomile oil
> 1 teaspoon vitamin E oil

Brew a small cup of chamomile tea and set aside to cool.

Combine the remaining ingredients in a small bowl and add the tea when completely cooled. Mix the ingredients well and pour into a small 300ml (10fl oz) pump bottle. Use within 1 month.

BODYWASH

Makes 75ml (2½fl oz)

> 3 tablespoons liquid Castile soap
> 2 tablespoons liquid carrier oil (any preferred)
> 10 drops essential oil of choice (or more if you prefer)

In a glass liquid measuring cup, carefully mix together all the ingredients with a spoon. Do not use a blender, whisk or handheld mixer as this will create bubbles and make it impossible to get it into a container.

Pour into a 75ml (2½fl oz) sterilized container and use in the shower as a body wash. I use with a natural sea sponge loofah.

This recipe will last for several months at room temperature.

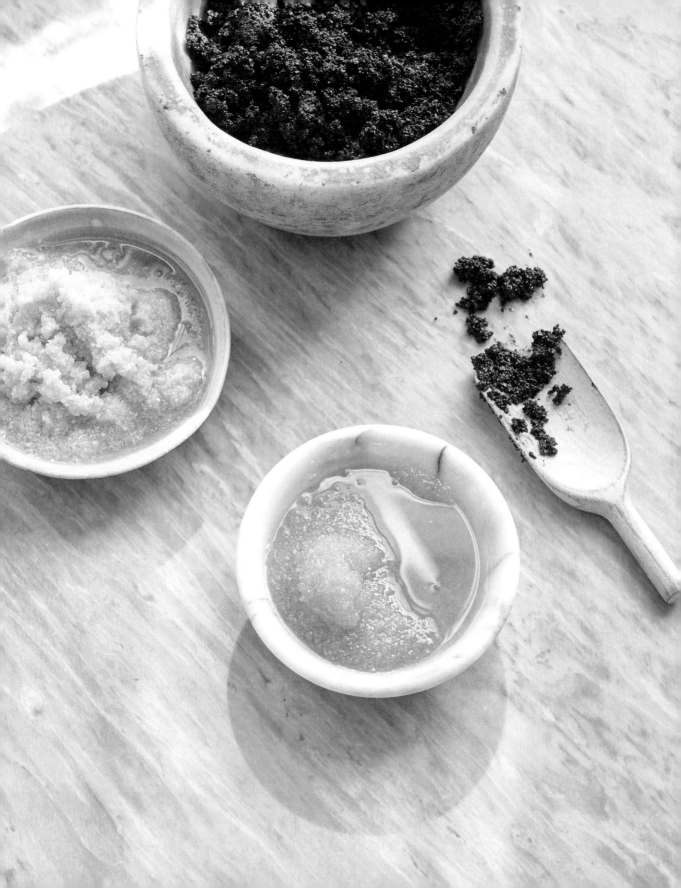

BODY *scrubs*

Sloughing away dead, flakey skin can be very beneficial, but it needs to be done gradually and gently. If the sting of salt feels too painful at first, try switching to sugar or coffee grounds. Always brush the scrub against your skin very lightly with the palm of your hand, and patch test on a small area first. If scrubbing your skin is too much right now, adding a handful of Dead Sea salts plus a cupful of oil to your bath is an alternative to reap those benefits.

Makes about 300g (10½oz)

COFFEE AND CINNAMON SCRUB

200g (7oz) coffee grounds
120ml (4fl oz) olive oil
1 teaspoon ground cinnamon
5 drops vanilla essential oil
5 drops sandalwood essential oil

Mix the ingredients together and transfer to a 300g (10½oz) sterilized jar. Use within 10–15 days.

SUGAR ALMOND SCRUB

200g (7oz) sugar (white or brown sugar is fine)
100ml (3½fl oz) sweet almond oil
1 tablespoon vitamin E oil
10 drops essential oil (choose your favourite)

Mix the ingredients together and transfer to a 300g (10½oz) sterilized jar. Use within 10–15 days.

DEAD SEA SALT SCRUB

200g (7oz) Dead Sea salt
100ml (3½fl oz) hemp seed oil
12 drops essential oil

Mix the ingredients together and transfer to a 300g (10½oz) sterilized jar. Use within 10–15 days.

OATMEAL *bath*

The simple soothing powers of oats are quite incredible! I would never have believed it myself had a sleepless night of itchy skin not led me to scour the internet for home remedies. That's where I first learned about oatmeal. Parents and doctors alike have been turning to the skin-soothing powers of oatmeal for centuries. It's not surprising, then, that you'll find colloidal oatmeal listed among the ingredients in many excellent natural body soaks, moisturizers and haircare products – I now use it in my own haircare range. Oatmeal is a natural way to lock in the body's moisture, protect the skin and soothe any irritation or itching.

Gentle enough to be used on delicate children's skin and ideal for even the most sensitive skin types, this simple bath soak is perfect for hydrating dry skin and offering relief from chronic skin conditions such as eczema.

Makes enough for 1 bath

100g (3½oz) oats – unflavoured instant oatmeal, quick oats or slow-cooking oats all work equally well

There are two ways to create your milky, soothing oatmeal bath. The first is to run your oats through a grinder or food-processor. Basically you want those oat flakes to transform into a fine powder, so that they can be readily absorbed into water without clumping or blocking the plug hole. Add a cupful to a warm water bath and soak for 15 minutes.

The second way, if you don't have a blender powerful enough to create a fine dust, is to simply add a couple of cups of oats to a muslin (cheesecloth) bag, tie the end and place it under the warm water while you run the bath.

Soak in the water for 15 minutes. You may even want to gently rub the muslin bag directly against your skin, if using the second method. Be careful getting in and out of the bath – oatmeal will make it even more slippery than usual.

Pat your skin dry with a super soft towel, and apply your favourite oil blend for extra hydration.

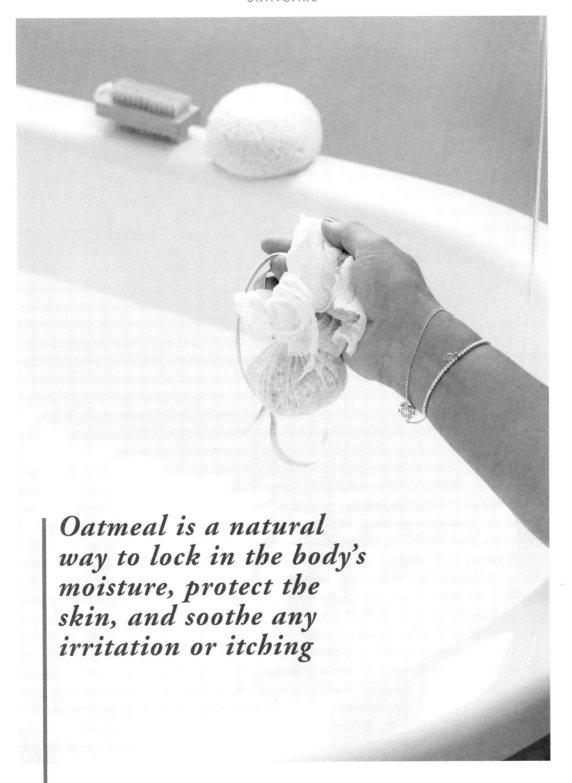

Oatmeal is a natural way to lock in the body's moisture, protect the skin, and soothe any irritation or itching

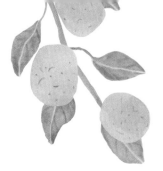

ACNE

I hated having my photo taken throughout high school. I was so shy at that time, and even though my psoriasis was well hidden with long sleeves, disguising acne on my face was virtually impossible. I tried every over-the-counter remedy I could find. Not one of them proved particularly effective. Part of my skin problem was definitely hormonal, but there was also something deeper going on and nothing seemed to resolve it. My doctor recommended a course of antibiotics, changing my birth control pill and trying strong prescription cleansers, but nothing worked. As a self-conscious teenager, I'd pretty much resigned myself to scarring from those spots and trowelling on thick foundation and concealer throughout my early twenties.

When it comes to hormone imbalance and our skin, this can feel like a particularly frustrating battle to resolve. That said, I've known people see dramatic improvements in their hormonal acne just through removing sugar and dairy products.

Going back to what we're learning about the microbiome, scientists are working on the theory that just as we have bacteria in the gut, we also have a microbiome in our mouths, on our skin and in other parts of the body. Emerging research suggests that probiotics and other substances that support the skin's microbiome can reduce inflammation, repair the skin barrier and reduce acne.

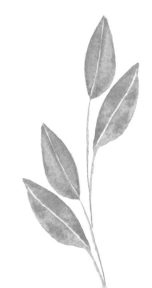

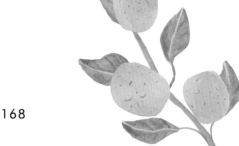

OIL *cleansers*

Oil cleansing uses a specific combination of oils to cleanse the skin and rebalance the skin's own natural oils, leaving it feeling nourished, hydrated and moisturized, where traditional soaps and synthetic cleaners can dry skin out. My favourite oil blends are below. Try different blends for yourself to find the one that best suits you. As we massage the cleansing oils into our skin, they dissolve oils that have hardened with impurities stuck in our pores. Using a hot steam cloth will open pores, allowing the stale oil to be easily removed.

As with any change to your skincare regime or diet, you might find you go through an adjustment period where skin briefly gets worse. It's mostly a detox reaction to impurities being pulled from the skin and should ease off in time.

Makes 100ml (3½fl oz)

FOR OILY SKIN
   30ml (2 tablespoons) castor oil
   70ml (4½ tablespoons) olive oil

FOR COMBINATION SKIN
   25ml (1½ tablespoons) hazelnut oil
   75ml (2½fl oz) hemp oil

FOR DRY SKIN
   90ml (3fl oz) olive oil
   10ml (2 teaspoons) hazelnut oil

Add your chosen blend to a 125ml (4fl oz) sterilized glass bottle and gently shake to combine. Shake again before each use. Store out of direct sunlight.

Pour a small quantity of oil into the palm of your hand and gently massage into dry skin for two minutes, or until you are sure that the oil has saturated your skin. This will also lift makeup very effectively, so there's no need to use harsh makeup removers. You can even leave the oil on the skin for up to 10 minutes to give pores a really deep clean.

Soak a clean wash cloth under a very hot tap. Wring it out and immediately place it over your face. The warmth of the water creates a lovely steamy effect, which works to remove dead skin cells and impurities clogged in pores. Leave the cloth on for a minute or two until it cools. Repeat if necessary with the opposite side of the wash cloth. There should still be a thin layer of oil remaining on the skin; this is beneficial and naturally moisturizing.

Your skin should feel hydrated, so you should not need any additional moisturizers, but if you still have especially dry skin, you might choose to massage in a small amount of homemade natural lotion. Use within 1 month.

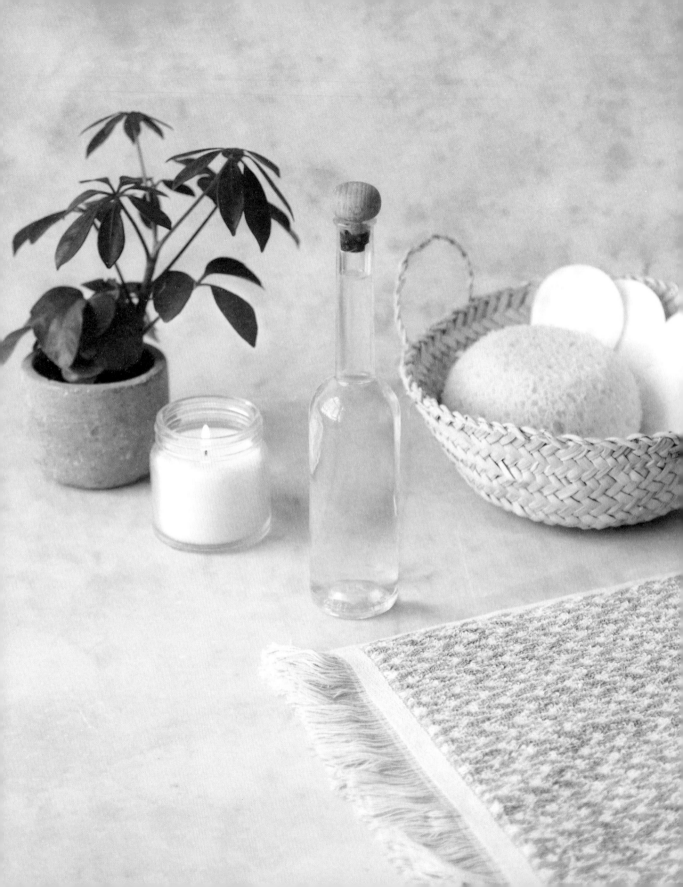

SEA SALT *soothing toner*

The minerals in Dead Sea salt can help to nourish skin, promoting a clear complexion. This soothing toner is ideal for acne-prone skin.

Makes 150ml (5fl oz)

1 tablespoon Dead Sea salt
Pinch of magnesium flakes
1–3 drops chamomile oil (optional)

Add the Dead Sea salt and magnesium flakes to 150ml (5fl oz) warm distilled water and stir until the salt has completely dissolved. Add the essential oil, if using, and store in a 150ml (5fl oz) sterilized glass bottle.

To use, apply to skin with a cotton pad as a toner. It's great for use as part of a daily skincare routine. Use within 1 month.

TEA TREE OIL *cleanser*

Tea tree oil has excellent disinfecting, soothing and antibacterial properties, so it's an excellent natural choice for treating acne. The oil penetrates our skin deeply, disinfecting the pores and drying out blackheads. This cleanser is made with just three simple ingredients.

Makes 325ml (11fl oz)

250m! (9fl oz) distilled water
75ml (2½fl oz) Castile liquid soap
15 drops tea tree oil

Carefully pour the distilled water and Castile soap into a 350ml (12fl oz) sterilized glass bottle with a pump. Add the drops of tea tree oil and shake together gently to combine. Use to cleanse your face in the morning and evenings. Store in the refrigerator for up to 1 month.

BENTONITE CLAY
mask

Bentonite clay can be used as an effective blackhead remover. It's known to contain more than 60 natural trace minerals such as calcium, iron, magnesium, potassium and silica, which make it an especially rich substance that has been used for centuries to treat a number of skin conditions. It's best for normal to oily skin, and has an electrical charge that actually helps remove toxins from the body. Bentonite clay removes toxins directly from the skin when applied topically, and also helps eliminate bacteria that can worsen blackheads.

Makes 1 treatment

1 tablespoon bentonite clay
Water or raw apple cider vinegar

Mix the bentonite clay with just enough water or raw apple cider vinegar to form a thick paste – it should be thick, but not so thick that it's clumpy or impossible to apply.

Wash your hands. Using your clean fingertips, apply a thin layer of paste to your face and allow it to sit for 10–15 minutes.

Rinse with lukewarm water and moisturize as you normally would.

BLACKHEADS

Blackheads are basically clogged pores, made up of dead skin cells and excess oils. While whiteheads are clogs in a closed pore, blackheads are clogs in an open pore (it's the exposure to air that turns the clog to a black colour).

Since blackheads are actually caused by oil in the skin – not dirt or other debris as you might think – washing the face too much can in fact cause more blackheads. Over washing your skin can dry it out and cause the sebaceous glands to produce too much oil. This might not be the only reason you're struggling with blackheads. Bacteria, hormonal changes and skin irritation can also be responsible.

CINNAMON *scrub*

Since blackheads are clogged pores, it's important to exfoliate the skin to reduce them. Over-the-counter exfoliators often include micro-beads and other synthetics that can cause environmental problems and can be especially harsh on sensitive skin.

Cinnamon is a wonderful scented spice that can eliminate flaky skin as well as acne, while bicarbonate of soda (baking soda) balances the skin's pH, encouraging it to stop producing excess oil.

Makes 1 treatment

½ **tablespoon ground cinnamon**
½ **teaspoon bicarbonate of soda (baking soda)**
1 **tablespoon coconut milk**

Mix the ingredients together into a smooth paste.

Wash your face with warm water and gently apply this mixture on your face in a circular motion. Focus on the areas with blackheads, like your nose and chin. The cinnamon will stick to the dirt in your pores and then pull it out as you sweep your fingers across your face.

Scrub for a couple of minutes, then wash your face clean with cold water and pat it dry.

It's important to exfoliate the skin to reduce blackheads

APPLE *skin toner*

Apple cider vinegar is a skin tonic that works very well in combatting blackheads and acne. It contains high amounts of acetic acid, which is great for our skin. It balances skin pH and tightens pores. It also has antibacterial, anti-inflammatory and antimicrobial properties, which help keep skin healthy.

   This toner recipe is intended for slightly oily skin. Witch hazel is a gentle astringent, apple cider vinegar will help restore your skin's natural pH balance and lavender soothes sensitive skin.

Makes 100ml (3½fl oz)

70ml (2½fl oz) witch hazel
30ml (1fl oz) raw apple cider vinegar
5 drops lavender essential oil

Pour all the ingredients into a 100ml (3½fl oz) sterilized spray bottle. Shake and use it as a regular facial toner.
   Store in the refrigerator for up to 1 month.

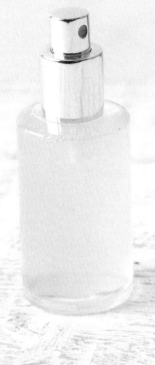

GREEN TEA *compress*

Green tea is loaded with anti-inflammatory and antioxidant properties and these have been proven to be beneficial in the treatment of rosacea. Cooled green tea can be applied as a compress, using a clean washcloth dipped in iced water.

Makes 1 treatment

3 green tea bags
700ml (1¼ pints) boiling water
Ice

In a bowl, soak the green tea bags in the boiling water, then refrigerate. When ready to use, remove the bowl from the refrigerator and add a handful of ice. Dip a clean cloth in the cooled green tea water and apply the compress to the affected area.

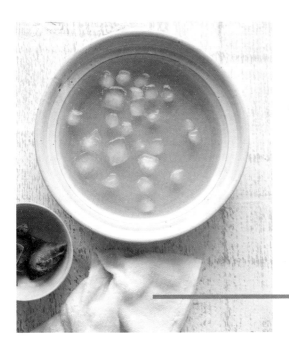

ROSACEA

Most conventional rosacea treatments include the use of oral and topical antibiotics. Drinking aloe vera water can help ease the symptoms of rosacea. It helps increase water content in the intestines, which in turn helps to eliminate toxins in the body, thereby reducing inflammation and lessening rosacea. Applying aloe vera gel, or using a green tea compress or colloidal oatmeal mask, can also help to relieve redness and inflammation.

EYELID *treatment*

Dermatitis on the eyelids causes them to become irritated, swollen, dry and red. This can affect one or both of the eyes. It's important to stop using soap, which can dry delicate skin out further. Restrict eye makeup use, which can also irritate the skin.

Makes 1

2–3 drops tea tree oil
1 tablespoon castor oil

Wash your eyelids and eyelashes thoroughly with lukewarm water. Apply a warm face cloth over the eyelids for 5 minutes.

Mix the tea tree oil with the castor oil. Dip two cotton wool balls in this solution. Close your eyes and dab a cotton ball on to your eyelids. Keep your eyes closed for 5–10 minutes. Repeat daily.

EXTRA GENTLE *aloe gel*

You might have applied aloe gel to sunburn in the past to cool the redness. Aloe penetrates the skin deeply and has soothing anti-inflammatory properties. This makes it great for use on skin conditions such as rosacea. It is possible to be sensitive or allergic to aloe vera, so always do a patch test before you apply it to larger areas.

Makes 135ml (4½fl oz)

125ml (4¼fl oz) aloe vera gel
2 tablespoons rosehip seed oil
3 drops lavender essential oil
2 drops chamomile essential oil
1 drop geranium essential oil

Combine the aloe vera gel and rose hip oil together, stirring well. Add the essential oils. Pour into a 150ml (5fl oz) glass bottle, preferably one with a pump action lid, and store in the refrigerator for 1 month.

Shake well before each use and apply twice daily.

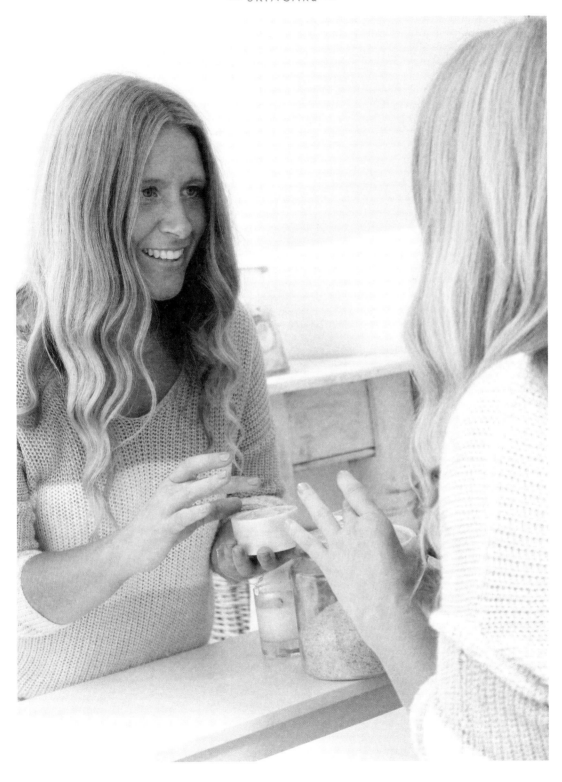

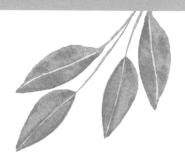

SCAR MINIMIZING

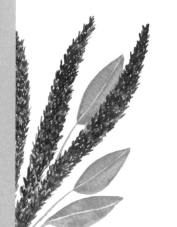

A scar is a mark left on the skin after a wound or injury has healed. Scars are a natural part of the healing process. Most will fade and become paler over time, although they never completely disappear.

Essential oils can discourage infection, encourage wounds to heal and decrease inflammation, which can all significantly assist in preventing scars from forming in the first place or help a scar's appearance to improve. You can dilute the following essentials oils for scars with a beneficial carrier oil. If you prefer a solid cream block, shea butter or coconut oil will work best. A good rule of thumb when diluting essential oils for adult use is a ratio of 2 per cent. That's 12 drops of essential oil, per 30ml (2 tablespoons) of carrier oil. If it comes to using scar minimizer on children's bumps and grazes, or if you have particularly sensitive skin, a ratio of 0.5 per cent would be my suggestion. To find out which carrier oil is most suited to your skin, see page 161.

SCAR MINIMIZING OILS

Rosehip – the vitamin C in rosehip oil can help reduce acne-related inflammation; the powerhouse ingredient boosts collagen and elastin production to encourage skin cell regeneration.

Vitamin E – this oil is an antioxidant, which means it can prevent oxidation and any damaging effects to the skin.

Geranium – this is useful in treating scars by relieving inflammation, evening out skin tone and encouraging new cell growth.

Cedar wood – this oil helps to clear out skin tissues that are not regenerating as fast as they should be and pulls out the excess fat that exists between tissues, which can also minimize the appearance of scars.

Frankincense – this oil is likely to improve the skin's repair process and decrease the chance of a scar forming.

Carrot seed – if you're looking for essential oils for scars and dark spot prevention, carrot seed oil may be a good choice.

HYPERPIGMENTATION *oil*

Carrot seed oil is not derived from the regular carrots we eat but from the wild carrot plant (botanical name: Daucus carota). It is actually a common roadside weed. It takes over three thousand seeds to squeeze out just one teaspoon of oil, which probably explains why it's one of the more expensive essential oils. Fortunately, this recipe only calls for a few drops.

Sandalwood encourages new cell formation and exfoliates the skin by removing dead cells, which in turn fades dark spots, blemishes and hyperpigmentation.

Makes about 60ml (2fl oz)

50ml (1¾fl oz) sesame oil
7 drops carrot seed oil
10 drops sandalwood oil

Using a small funnel, pour the sesame oil into a 60ml (2fl oz) sterilized amber glass dropper bottle. Now add the essential oils, drop by drop.

Close the bottle and shake gently to combine all oils. Store in a cool dry place and use within 2 months.

To use, gently massage 2–4 drops onto your skin before bedtime.

HYPERPIGMENTATION

Hyperpigmentation is the term used to describe darker areas of uneven pigmentation in skin. Post-inflammatory hyper-pigmentation occurs when a skin injury or trauma heals and leaves a flat area of discolouration behind. It's caused by an increase in melanin, the natural pigment that gives our skin, hair and eyes their colour. A number of factors can trigger this increase in melanin production, but the main ones are sun exposure, hormonal influences, age and skin injuries or inflammation.

ANTI-ITCH *spray*

Makes 50ml (1¾fl oz)

2 tablespoons witch hazel
1 teaspoon Dead Sea salt
Pinch of menthol crystals
1 tablespoon aloe vera gel
1 teaspoon raw apple cider vinegar
2–3 drops lavender essential oil
2–3 drops calendula essential oil

Pour the witch hazel into a glass bowl, then place on top of a pan of boiling water.

Add 1 teaspoon of the sea salt and a pinch of the menthol crystals. Stir well until the ingredients blend completely.

Add the aloe vera gel and raw apple cider vinegar. Add 2–3 drops each of lavender and calendula essential oils. Mix everything well and funnel the liquid into a 60ml (2fl oz) sterilized amber spray bottle.

Simply spray the solution on irritated or itchy skin to get instant relief. Reapply as needed.

Store the spray in a dark, cool place or the refrigerator. The shelf life is 1–2 weeks if you use fresh aloe vera gel from the plant. If you use packaged gel, the spray should stay good for 2–3 months.

SOOTHING *lotion*

Makes 75ml (2½fl oz)

60ml (2fl oz) olive oil
1 tablespoon shea butter
3 tablespoons coconut oil
1 tablespoon sunflower wax pellets
10 drops frankincense essential oil
10 drops lavender essential oil
5 drops peppermint essential oil

Place the olive oil, shea butter, coconut oil and sunflower wax pellets in a glass bowl over a pan filled with water. Heat the water to warm the ingredients, while stirring, as they melt. Continue to stir until well blended. Remove from the heat and stir in the essential oils. Allow it to cool and check the consistency.

Place in a 100ml (3½fl oz) sterilized container. Apply, as needed, to soothe irritation. Store in the refrigerator for up to 1 month.

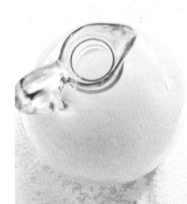

SOOTHING SKIN *mask*

Itchy and particularly aggravated skin can be incredibly frustrating to live with. This six-ingredient mask can help provide effective and soothing relief from itching that has been brought on not only by long-term skin conditions, but also by temporary flares from stings, bites, chickenpox and allergy rashes.

Makes 75ml (2½fl oz)

- 1 tablespoon bentonite clay
- 1 tablespoon pink kaolin clay
- 1 tablespoon bicarbonate of soda (baking soda)
- 1 tablespoon Dead Sea salt
- 1 tablespoon raw apple cider vinegar
- 5 drops lavender essential oil

Combine the bentonite and pink kaolin clays, bicarbonate of soda, sea salt and raw apple cider vinegar with enough water to make a creamy paste. Add the lavender essential oil and mix well.

Store in a 75ml (2½fl oz) sterilized glass container with a non-metal lid in the refrigerator for several weeks. Apply to stings, bites, rashes and skin irritations as needed. Allow to dry each time you apply it, then rinse off with warm water.

Warning Use non-metal bowls, utensils and storage containers for this project. Metal can react with the ingredients causing them to lose their effectiveness.

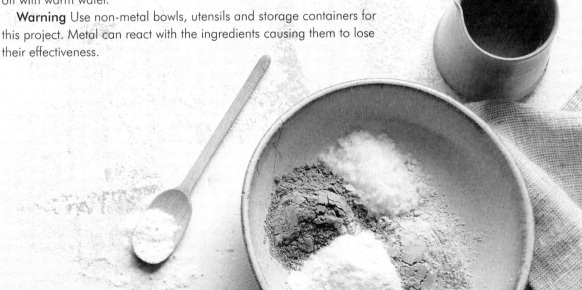

OATMEAL *mask*

Oatmeal is a wonderful natural moisturizer and an excellent exfoliator. You can prepare an oatmeal mask when required to leave the skin feeling hydrated and intensely nourished.

Makes 1 treatment

50g (1¾oz) oatmeal, powdered (you can grind it in a coffee bean grinder or blender)

Put the powdered oatmeal in a bowl and gradually keep adding water to make a smooth paste. Apply it to the skin and let it completely dry for 5–10 minutes.

Splash water on to your face to rehydrate the mask, then rub gently to exfoliate. Wash the mask off fully with warm water.

SEA SALT *spray*

Those of us struggling with psoriasis and eczema often see improvements in our skin at the beach. It makes sense: between a combination of vitamin D and the magnesium and minerals in the water, the beach can be great for skin health. For those of us who don't live near the ocean, this homemade spray can help achieve some of those same awesome benefits at home.

Makes 250ml (8½fl oz)

3 tablespoons dried calendula petals
250ml (8½fl oz) simmering water
1 tablespoon Dead Sea salt
1 teaspoon magnesium flakes
1–3 drops essential oil of choice
   (optional)

Place the calendula flowers in a mug and pour the simmering hot water over them.

Put the salt and magnesium into a bowl. Sieve the calendula water and pour the infused water over the salt. Discard the petals. Stir until the salt is completely dissolved. Allow to cool.

Add your favourite essential oils, if using, and store in a 300ml (10fl oz) sterilized glass jar or spray bottle. Apply to skin by spraying liberally. Store out of direct sunlight for up to 1 month.

VITAMIN C
swim spray

I absolutely love swimming. I most definitely think I was a mermaid in another life. My skin, however, has other ideas. While it seems to love the salt in the ocean, I really struggle with chlorinated water. I have a fantastic open air pool close to me that I enjoy swimming in all year round, but unfortunately they use chlorine. I use this spray right before my swim and afterward just after showering. It really works to neutralize chlorine exposure on the body.

There are two types of vitamin C, both of which can neutralize chlorine – sodium ascorbate and ascorbic acid. While either version will work in this recipe, I prefer sodium ascorbate. It's less acidic and won't lower the skin's pH like ascorbic acid can. It also dissolves more easily, making it easier to mix.

While I would almost always recommend storing skincare products in amber glass, this particular recipe is much safer in a plastic bottle with a spray cap. You definitely don't want any breakages around swimming pools or communal showers.

Makes 265ml (9fl oz)

200ml (7fl oz) fractionated coconut oil
1 teaspoon vitamin C powder
2 tablespoons magnesium oil
2 tablespoons Dead Sea salt
5 drops frankincense essential oil

Add all the ingredients to a 300ml 10fl oz) sterilized plastic bottle and shake well. Store in a cool, dark place for up to 1 month.

HOMEMADE
eyeshadow

The shea butter helps create a soft, creamy powder that stays on and moisturizes eyelids at the same time, though it still has a powdery texture. I use a mortar bowl and pestle to help blend ingredients. If you want a lighter eyeshadow, use a little more arrowroot powder. It's easy to keep adding as you go, so starting with less will offer more flexibility in your recipe. Arrowroot has anti-inflammatory properties and is historically known to heal wounds.

Makes 10g (^{1}/$_3$oz)

½ teaspoon arrowroot powder
1 teaspoon colour combination (see below)
1 teaspoon shea butter

In a small mortar bowl, place the arrowroot powder. Add your chosen colour combination, starting with a small amount, then adding more, blending well.

Add a little shea butter to the mixture. You can use the back of a spoon or a pestle to blend it well. The mixture will still be powdery. Place in a small, clean makeup container.

Apply a small amount to clean eyelids using a cotton swab or an eyeshadow brush applicator. Use within 2 weeks.

COLOUR COMBINATIONS

Brown – cacao powder, ground cinnamon or ground nutmeg
Golden – ground turmeric
Pink – beetroot or hibiscus powder
Green – matcha or spirulina
Black/Grey – activated charcoal
Orange – saffron and beetroot powder
To lighten or darken – white, red or rose clays can be used lighten or darken the colour
Glitter – micas can be used for glitter and a shimmery sparkle

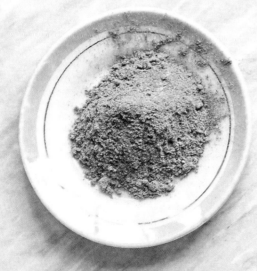
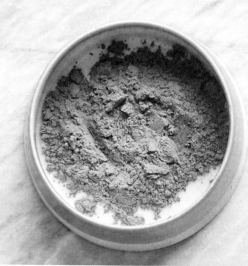

HOMEMADE *blush*

The quantity of ingredients you actually use will vary by skin tone. There might be a little trial and error to begin with, and you'll have to experiment with small amounts of each powder to blend the shade that works for you.

Makes 10g ($^1/_3$oz)

½ teaspoon arrowroot powder
½ teaspoon cacao powder
½ teaspoon hibiscus or beetroot powder
½ teaspoon ground nutmeg

Start with a base of ½ teaspoon of arrowroot and darken with the other ingredients as needed. When you get your desired shade, store in a small, clean airtight jar or old makeup shaker and use as blush. Use within 1 month.

LIP *gloss*

Makes 30ml (1fl oz)

½ teaspoon sunflower wax pellets
1 teaspoon shea butter
1 teaspoon fractionated coconut oil
4 teaspoons castor oil
5 drops your favourite essential oil (for flavour)
Red pigment, such as beetroot powder

Place all the ingredients, except the essential oils and red powder, into a glass bowl over a saucepan of simmering water. Once melted, remove from the heat and cool for a couple of minutes.

Add your chosen essential oil and a pinch of powder, then stir until combined. Start with just a little and add more until you get the desired colour.

Carefully pour your gloss into small, clean 15ml (½fl oz) containers and pop in the refrigerator to set. Use within 2 weeks.

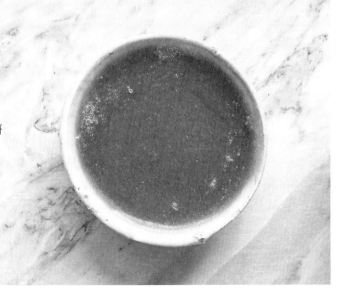

MAKE *a plan*

Thinking about the five elements of gut healing we've spoken about, it's time to make your plan. It's not compulsory to add something to every single section. It might be that you're not ready to work on certain aspects just yet, or maybe there are bits of the jigsaw that are already in place for you. The key is to tailor a protocol that works for you, focusing on the parts that need extra input. Decide exactly what you're going to commit to each week, implement those changes and ultimately strengthen your circle of wellbeing.

	WEEK ONE	WEEK TWO	WEEK THREE	WEEK FOUR
DIET				
MIND				
EXERCISE				
SLEEP				
SKINCARE				

LONG *run*

Thinking about your longer-term goals, what would you like to achieve in the future? This is a good space to consider bigger life changes. Whether it's transitioning to a completely vegan diet, going on a yoga retreat, completing a marathon. Dream big and set your intentions.

DIET

MIND

EXERCISE

SLEEP

SKINCARE

TEN POINT *plan*

1. Eat a healthy, plant-based diet full of fruit, vegetables, nuts and seeds, avoiding meat, wheat, dairy, nightshades and refined sugar.

2. Hydrate well by eliminating or reducing caffeine and alcohol. Drink 2–3 litres (3½–5¼ pints) of still water per day, plus herbal teas.

3. Juice! Flood your body with liquid nutrients.

4. Move your body. Whether with gentle yoga or intensive cardio, get your lymphatic system moving on a regular basis.

5. Work on stress levels and anxiety through mindfulness and meditation.

6. Practice gratitude daily. Focus on the positive elements in your life.

7. Draw up a bedtime routine and create a restful environment to consistently get a good night's sleep.

8. Ditch toxic skincare in favour of beneficial natural botanicals that will nourish your skin, not strip it of its natural oils.

9. Celebrate the small stuff. Don't forget to acknowledge your achievements along the way.

10. Don't be afraid to reach out for guidance. Similarly, once you're further along your healing path, share your story to help inspire others and continue to grow our empowering skin-healing community.

acknowledgements

What a whirlwind the past three years have been. I can't believe so much time has gone by since we published Radiant. As a debut author, I was incredibly nervous publishing my first book, but the response it's received and the amazing before-and-after photographs I get sent each week from people inspired to follow my plan make me so proud. In that time, our online healing community has grown stronger, warriors have told their amazing stories on my podcast, I've spoken at food and wellness festivals around the country and shared one of the most incredible experiences of my life – appearing on Dragons' Den! Bringing my skincare range and this second book to life since the show has been the icing on the cake.

It has been a very personal journey, but I could not have done it without the incredible support of lots of people working tirelessly behind the scenes. Those who very much believed in my vision and clearly understood my passion for helping people struggling with their skin. To Ollie, Ian, Chloe, Carmel and the team who helped me formulate my amazing skincare range. To Grace, who not only illustrated the skincare range so beautifully but also worked on the gorgeous illustrations in this book. To Simon, for helping me keep calm and confident. To Kris, for making sure I didn't mess up the numbers. To Tej and his brilliant team, especially Stepan and Charles. To Peter and his fantastic team, especially John. I've learned so much since the Den and I'm excited to continue that journey.

To everyone involved in creating this beautiful book, especially Paula, Caroline, Danielle and Kate, for openly sharing their very personal healing stories. To Judith, for allowing me to continue sharing my own healing journey with the world. To Megan and the food styling team, for presenting each meal to look utterly delicious. To my talented photographer Clare, who effortlessly captured these beautiful food and skincare recipes. To Tania, for once again creating a design I just love. To Tara, my brilliant editor, who has been immensely patient, making everything appear all graceful and swan-like on the surface, whilst at times I've felt as though I'm furiously paddling my feet beneath the water! And to my agent Becky, who has worked brilliantly hard to look after me, as always.

Finally, to my online skin-healing community, my family and friends, both here in the UK and dotted around the world. Thank you for being so brilliantly kind. For sharing my excitement through the fun times and supporting me with words, hugs and patience through the more difficult moments. I feel very blessed and thankful that you're a part of my journey.